Essentials in Cytopathology

Series Editor
Dorothy L. Rosenthal

More information about this series at
http://www.springer.com/series/6996

Yener S. Erozan • Armanda Tatsas

Cytopathology of Liver, Biliary Tract, Kidney and Adrenal Gland

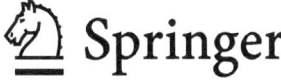 Springer

Yener S. Erozan
Department of Pathology
The Johns Hopkins University
    School of Medicine
Baltimore, MD, USA

Armanda Tatsas
Pathology Group of Louisiana
Baton Rouge, LA, USA

ISSN 1574-9053   ISSN 1574-9061 (electronic)
ISBN 978-1-4899-7512-6   ISBN 978-1-4899-7513-3 (eBook)
DOI 10.1007/978-1-4899-7513-3
Springer New York Heidelberg Dordrecht London

Library of Congress Control Number: 2014949164

Printed on acid-free paper

Springer is part of Springer Science+Business Media (www.springer.com)

To Brenda

— Yener S. Erozan

To Alon, Natasha, and Sarah,
for teaching me something new every day

— Armanda Tatsas

Preface

Percutaneous and endoscopic ultrasound (EUS)-guided fine needle aspirations have been used widely in the diagnosis of intraabdominal lesions detected by imaging studies. These are safe, highly accurate, and minimally invasive techniques. Because FNA diagnosis also can aid in the selection of the type of therapy (surgical vs. nonsurgical) in some cases, high accuracy is critical. This can be achieved by teamwork between the radiologist (or other physician performing the FNA) and the pathologist. Collection of adequate specimens, proper preparation of the material, and the pathologist's experience are obvious factors in reaching the correct diagnosis.

In *Fine Needle Aspirations of Liver, Kidney and Adrenal Glands*, the percutaneous approach is usually used. In recent literature, however, EUS-guided FNAs of these organs have been reported. The first chapter of the book, written by radiologists Dr. Stephanie Coquia and Dr. Ulrike M. Hamper, presents key clinical and technical features of image guidance methods for FNA of intraabdominal masses and organs. On-site evaluation, discussed in the second chapter, assures that adequate specimens are obtained and determines whether the specimen should be sent for special studies, e.g., flow cytometry. In the organ-specific chapters, although emphasis is on the cytomorphology of the lesions, additional studies, such as immunohistochemical stains in cell blocks or core biopsies, are presented as needed for the specific diagnosis.

This book is meant to be a practical guide for the diagnosis of lesions, mostly neoplasms, of liver, kidney, and adrenal glands. We believe that the cytopathologic diagnosis of malignancy should be made cautiously after careful examination of the material, and it should be as accurate as a tissue diagnosis.

Baltimore, MD, USA   Yener S. Erozan, M.D.
Baton Rouge, LA, USA   Armanda Tatsas, M.D.

Contents

Contributors

Stephanie F. Coquia, M.D. Department of Radiology and Radiological Science, Johns Hopkins Outpatient Center, Johns Hopkins Medical Institutions, Baltimore, MD, USA

Yener S. Erozan, M.D. Department of Pathology, The Johns Hopkins University, School of Medicine, Baltimore, MD, USA

Ulrike M. Hamper, M.D. Department of Radiology and Radiological Science, Johns Hopkins Hospital, Baltimore, MD, USA

Armanda Tatsas, M.D. Pathology Group of Louisiana, Baton Rouge, LA, USA

Chapter 1
Image-Guided Fine Needle Aspiration of Intra-abdominal Masses and Organs: Liver, Kidney, and Adrenal Gland

Stephanie F. Coquia and Ulrike M. Hamper

Indications

Image-guided percutaneous fine needle aspiration (FNA) biopsy is a safe, cost-effective, and time efficient method of biopsy. In most instances, it has replaced open surgical biopsy. There are several indications for fine needle aspiration. Broadly, they are performed to confirm malignancy in a suspicious lesion, diagnose an indeterminate lesion, or confirm a probably benign lesion. The clinical question to be answered is whether the lesion is a metastasis, a primary malignancy, or benign. Diagnosing the lesion correctly has important implications for patient treatment. Confirming a lesion is metastatic

S.F. Coquia, M.D. (✉)
Department of Radiology and Radiological Science, Johns Hopkins Outpatient Center, Johns Hopkins Medical Institutions, 601 N. Caroline Street Suite 3142, Baltimore, MD 21287, USA
e-mail: scoquia1@jhmi.edu

U.M. Hamper, M.D.
Department of Radiology and Radiological Science, Johns Hopkins Hospital, Sheikh Zayed Tower, 1800 Orleans Street Suite 4030, Baltimore, MD 21287, USA
e-mail: umhamper@jhu.edu

Y.S. Erozan and A. Tatsas, *Cytopathology of Liver, Biliary Tract, Kidney and Adrenal Gland*, Essentials in Cytopathology 18, DOI 10.1007/978-1-4899-7513-3_1,
© Springer Science+Business Media New York 2015

rather than a primary malignancy may direct the patient toward chemotherapy or radiation therapy rather than surgery. In addition, recent advances in molecular imaging and novel treatment methods of tumors through individual genetic markers or vaccine therapies have increased the demand on FNA and core biopsies. Please see the section "Specific Anatomic Applications" regarding organ-specific indications for biopsy. Furthermore, FNA can be performed to assess parenchymal disease in native organs such as liver and kidney or in renal, hepatic, and pancreas transplants.

Contraindications

There are very few contraindications to image-guided FNA due to its minimally invasive approach. An uncorrectable bleeding disorder or lack of a safe path to target the mass may preclude the biopsy. A cooperative patient is key to the success of the biopsy. As the liver, kidney, and adrenal gland move during breathing, the patient's ability to hold their breath is important in the targeting and successful sampling of the mass during fine needle aspiration.

Complications

Again, due to its minimally invasive approach, there are relatively few complications, and serious complications are rare. Minor complications include a vasovagal reaction or pain. Infection is a rare complication, especially if sterile technique is used. Bleeding is a risk, but typically a small hematoma may be the most that occurs. Damage to adjacent organs, including the lung and diaphragm, is also a rare complication. The more serious complications, bleeding and damage to adjacent organs, are minimized by image guidance and patient cooperation during the procedure. As these procedures are performed in the imaging suite, these complications can be swiftly diagnosed and treated. Needle track seeding is uncommon.

Patient Preparation

Typically a preprocedure call is made to the patient. The procedure requires fasting in the event a serious complication requiring intubation occurs. Up to date laboratory work is requested and reviewed, typically including a check of platelets, prothrombin time with international normalized ratio (PT/INR), and partial thromboplastin time (PTT). Review of the patient's medications is also performed, with any medications affecting the patient's clotting ability held for at least several days prior to the procedure. Every service has its own set of guidelines for what is acceptable for biopsy. These guidelines also depend on the organ to be targeted, with deep or very vascular organs requiring stricter adherence to a normal coagulation profile.

On the day of the biopsy, the performing physician will obtain informed consent and assess the patient's status. The vast majority of these procedures can be performed under local anesthesia, but some patients may require a small dose of an anxiolytic or analgesic. Rarely a patient will require conscious sedation, either by the performing physician and nurse or by anesthesia. Rarely is general anesthesia required, except in small children. Assistance from the anesthesia team should be prearranged.

Based on the approach of the procedure, the patient may be placed in the prone, supine, lateral decubitus, or even semierect position. The biopsy team will assess the lesion under imaging to plan for the needle approach and also to assess the lesion's movement with the patient's breathing. If breath holding is required, a few practice breath-holds with the patient are performed to ensure optimal patient cooperation during the procedure.

Image Guidance Methods

The two main methods of image guidance are via ultrasound (US) or computed tomography (CT). Magnetic resonance imaging (MRI) Rarely is magnetic resonance imaging (MR)

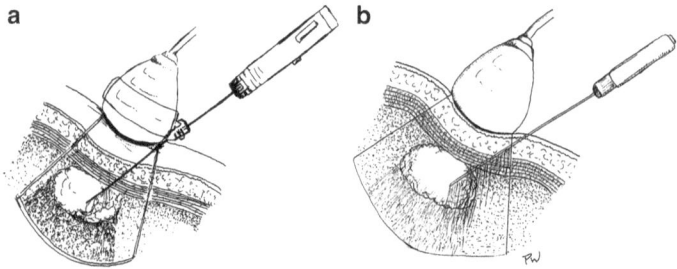

FIG. 1.1.   (**a**) Schematic showing guide attached to ultrasound probe for guided technique. The guide controls the angulation of the needle. (**b**) Schematic showing free hand technique (without guide). The operator controls the angulation of the needle. Images courtesy of Paul Wiernicki, RDMS, RVT.

guidance is used rarely; when a lesion can only be visualized with this modality. The advantages and limitations of US and CT techniques are described below. When choosing a modality, one must assess the modality's ability to image the lesion adequately, the size of the lesion, the equipment availability, and the performing physician's own facility with it.

Ultrasound Guidance

Ultrasound allows for real time visualization of the needle as well as the target during biopsy. The capillary action of the needle during fine needle aspiration can be watched on the ultrasound monitor to confirm correct sampling. There are unlimited scan planes depending on the patient's positioning and the positioning of the probe. A guide can be attached to the probe in order to direct the needle correctly to the lesion along a predetermined and controlled path (Fig. 1.1a). However, some operators may choose to perform a "freehand" technique, where instead of the guide controlling the degree of angulation of the needle, the operator may do so instead. This technique allows the operator additional flexibility in approach; however, this technique is more difficult to learn and teach and is more time consuming (Fig. 1.1b). Color Doppler can be used to visualize vessels that should be avoided. In a mass of a substantial size, Color Doppler can be used to assess for viable tissue (areas of increased vascularity) that may yield a better sample for pathology. Ultrasound is also portable, has lower cost, and no radiation. However, performing a procedure under ultrasound guidance requires expertise on the part of the physician (with or without the help of a sonographer) to find the lesion, hold the probe, direct the patient's breathing, and perform the biopsy simultaneously.

Knowledge of the lesion's location on CT or MR is used to target the lesion under US. If the lesion is difficult to see under ultrasound independently, ultrasound machines with fusion imaging capability can be used. CT and MR images from a patient's prior study can be imported into the machine's computer and fused with real-time ultrasound images to localize a lesion (Fig. 1.2).

CT Guidance

To some extent, the actual needle insertion is performed blind to minimize radiation to the patient and to the performing physician as well as to minimize artifacts from motion and from the needle. CT can be used to determine THE depth and angulation of the needle NEEDED to reach the lesion. A CT scanner equipped with CT fluoroscopy where the operator may direct the radiation to a small set of axial slices (typically three) centered around the target may be helpful in directing/redirecting the needle along the right path to the lesion. Sampling of the lesion once the target has been reached is also performed blindly with the patient outside of the CT gantry. Most CT fine needle aspirations are performed using a coaxial approach with an introducer, therefore trying to sample different areas within the INTRODUCER can be difficult.

Endoscopic Guidance

Gastroenterologists using endoscopic ultrasound perform this procedure. An ultrasound probe is attached to the endoscope. Although fine needle aspiration via endoscopic ultrasound is

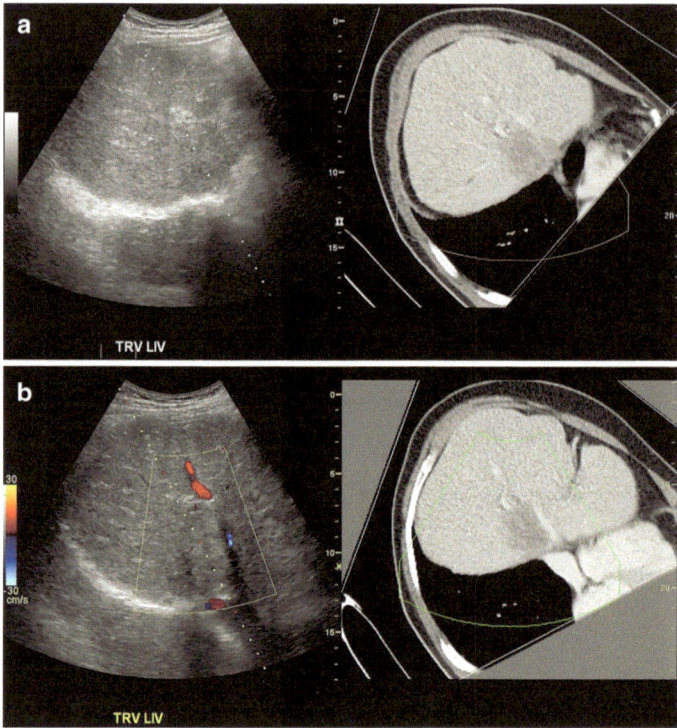

FIG. 1.2.   (**a**) Use of CT images to localize lesion under ultrasound with fusion technique. (**b**) Second image shows fusion plus color Doppler, to show absence of large central hepatic blood vessels in the path of the biopsy. Pathology of the lesion was moderately differentiated adenocarcinoma. Note the *dotted line* on the image, denoting the projected path of the biopsy needle.

used commonly today in the diagnosis of pancreatic tumors, expanding the technique to other organs has only happened fairly recently. Based on proximity of the lesion to the gastrointestinal tract, endoscopic ultrasound can only visualize lesions in the left hepatic lobe, left kidney, and left adrenal gland. This technique is being performed only at certain centers across the country. In contrast to US-guided FNAs, endoscopic procedures are more invasive and time consuming and require deep sedation.

Biopsy Technique

The most important part of the procedure is the planning of the approach. Once the imaging modality has been chosen, the target visualized, the tract planned, and the patient is comfortable, the procedure may begin.

The area on the skin where the needle will enter is marked. The skin is cleaned with Betadine or more preferably with ChloraPrep® (2 % Chlorhexidine Gluconate/70 % Isopropyl Alcohol) because of its faster action and broader spectrum to fight bacteria. The site is covered with sterile drapes or towels to keep a sterile field. One percent buffered lidocaine is used for local anesthesia. A small wheal is made under the skin. Once the skin is numb, deeper anesthesia is applied under imaging guidance. The liver has a capsule with nerve endings that are irritated by the biopsy which, when breached by the needle, may cause the patient pain. It is the site of the deeper anesthesia for liver biopsies. For the kidney and adrenal gland, anesthesia is introduced to the level of the lesion and along its tract.

Once deeper anesthesia has been achieved, the biopsy portion may begin. If the biopsy is performed under CT guidance, an introducer is placed into the lesion for a coaxial approach. Similarly, a guide is placed on the ultrasound probe to direct the needle to the target. Once the lesion is reached, the stylette is removed and the needle is moved in a swift, repetitive, up and down motion in the lesion. This capillary action allows the cells to be drawn up into the needle. The needle is then removed from the target, and the cells are placed on the slide for pathology. Sometimes, and particularly in a very fibrous lesion, aspiration via an attached syringe is necessary to obtain sufficient material.

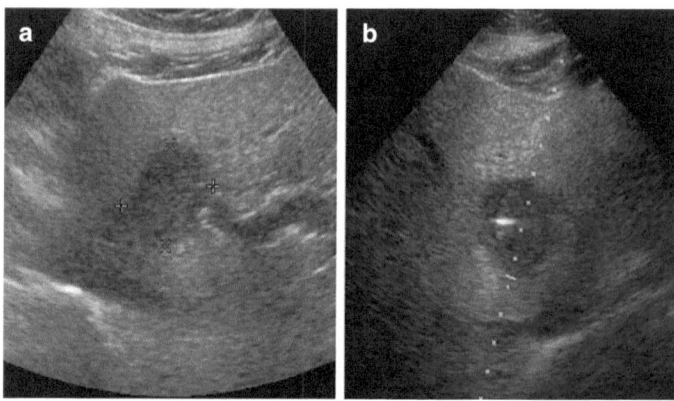

FIG. 1.3.   (**a** and **b**) Hypoechoic lesion in the liver (between calipers) allows for better visualization of THE needle tip within the lesion as seen in **b**. Pathology of the lesion was metastatic breast cancer.

Typically core needle biopsies are requested at the time of the biopsy, and these can be performed using the same approach as the fine needle aspiration.

Needle Selection and Visualization

The most common needles used for fine needle aspiration are 22 gauge Chiba or spinal needles which come in a variety of lengths. Occasionally, 25 or 20 gauge needles can be used. In many cases a renal lesion, particularly one suspected of being a renal cell carcinoma, may yield only blood on fine needle aspiration with a 22 gauge needle. A smaller gauge may create fewer traumas and bleeding and yield more diagnostic material. Core biopsies are typically performed with larger gauge needles: 20, 18, or even 16 gauges.

Despite using ultrasound guidance and a guide, the needle may be difficult to see. The needle is best seen when the lesion in question is hypoechoic (Fig. 1.3). The more echogenic the lesion is, the more difficult it is to see the needle, as the needle itself is hyperechoic. Needles with serrated tips may be better visualized. A few techniques may be performed to increase visualization of the needle: rock the transducer slowly back and forth, bob the needle or stylette, insert a trace of air, or use the color artifact created by motion on Color Doppler US.

On-site Pathologic Evaluation

On-site evaluation for adequacy of the specimen is performed by a pathologist in all image-guided fine needle aspirations. Details of the procedure are discussed in Chap. 2.

Specific Anatomic Applications

Liver

The liver is the most common site of biopsy within the abdomen. The usual indication for a liver biopsy is a patient with either one lesion or multiple lesions who has a known primary tumor. Although by imaging they may appear as metastases, tissue confirmation is needed to stage the lesion prior to treatment of the primary tumor or for further characterization by immunohistochemistry and molecular markers. Another scenario may be a patient with multiple lesions without any known or radiographically visible underlying disease. The tissue from the biopsy may be used to determine the source of the primary tumor. The appearance of hepatic abscesses and metastases may also overlap, so a biopsy may be performed to distinguish between the two pathologies. Lastly, another frequent indication for biopsy is a patient with cirrhosis who has a lesion or lesions that could reflect hepatocellular carcinoma (Fig. 1.4). In addition, assessment for parenchymal disease in native or transplanted livers is made through large gauge (typically 18 gauge) core biopsies.

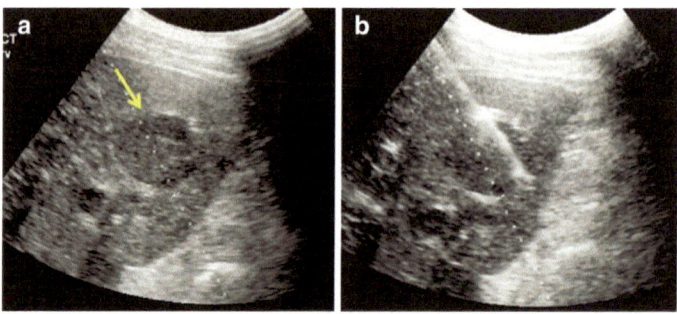

FIG. 1.4. (**a**) Hypoechoic liver lesion (*arrow*) biopsied with use of needle guide. (**b**) Shorten to biopsy needle traversing the lesion. Pathology of the lesion was hepatocellular carcinoma. The underlying liver had a coarsened echotexture, which can be seen in cirrhosis.

Kidney

Typically, suspicious renal masses are excised with nephrectomy, partial nephrectomy, or treated with radiofrequency or cryo-ablation. However, occasionally a request for FNA is received. In many of those cases, the patient has an underlying malignancy and the renal mass may represent a metastasis, a second primary tumor, or lymphoma. Based on the results of the biopsy, this patient may be directed toward chemotherapy rather than surgery. Alternatively, the patient may not be a surgical candidate and tissue is needed prior to the start of chemotherapy. Some lesions, such as atypical cystic renal masses, are indeterminate on imaging, and biopsy may determine whether the patient can be managed conservatively or should be sent to surgery (Fig. 1.5). In addition, assessment for parenchymal disease in native or transplanted kidneys is made through large gauge (typically 18 gauge) core biopsies.

Adrenal Gland

The most common indication for biopsy of the adrenal gland is to confirm metastatic disease or differentiate metastatic disease from a primary adrenal lesion such as adenoma or

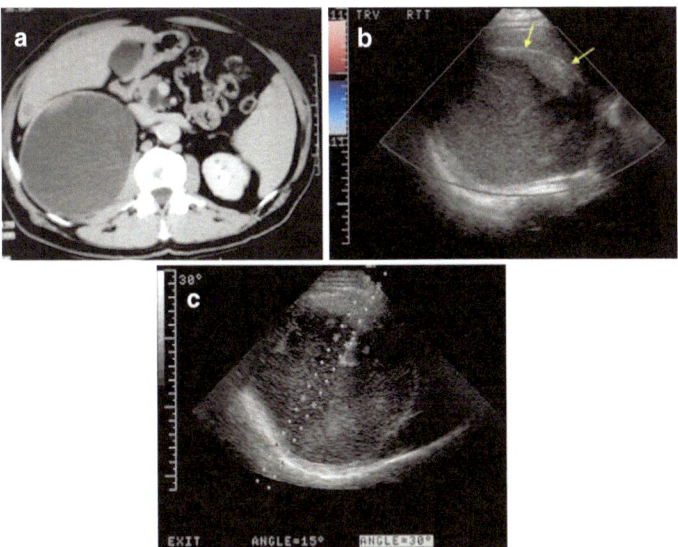

Fig. 1.5. (**a**) Cystic renal lesion within the right kidney on CT showing a soft tissue component along the anterior lateral aspect of the lesion. (**b**) Corresponding appearance on US showing the anterior soft tissue component, which should be targeted for biopsy (*arrows*). (**c**) US-guided biopsy of anterior soft tissue component.

adrenal carcinoma. Due to its relatively small size compared to the liver and kidney and its retroperitoneal location, the approach may be different than for a liver or kidney lesion. The right adrenal gland may have to be reached via a transhepatic or posterior approach (Fig. 1.6). The left adrenal gland may have to be accessed via an anterior, lateral, or posterior/oblique approach (Fig. 1.7). A transpleural or transpancreatic approach should be avoided due to the increased risk of complications. Biopsy of a pheochromocytoma is also to be avoided because of the potential of a hypertensive crisis when inadvertently biopsied, unless the patient is adequately premedicated with alpha-adrenergic blockers and metyrosine.

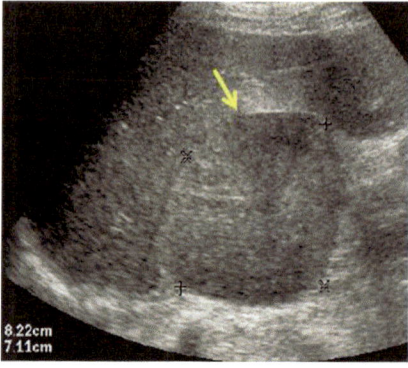

FIG. 1.6.   Large right adrenal lesion (*arrow*) adjacent to the liver, requiring a transhepatic approach. The pathology was metastatic endometrial cancer.

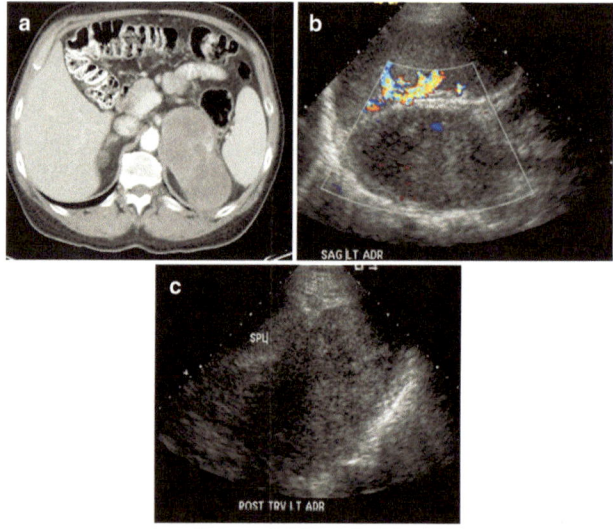

FIG. 1.7.   (**a**) CT showing large left adrenal mass. (**b**) US showing anterior approach, which would require going through the spleen and its hilum, which should be avoided. (**c**) US showing posterior approach, which would avoid the spleen. The approach was chosen for biopsy. The pathology was compatible with metastasis. *SPL* spleen.

Other Issues

As with any fine needle aspiration procedure, needle safety is imperative in protecting all members of the medical team from injury. Acute awareness at all times of the placement of needles, particularly those containing body fluids, is important for pathologists and cytotechnologists performing on-site evaluation.

Conclusions

Image-guided percutaneous FNA is a safe, cost-effective, and time efficient alternative to open surgical biopsy. Like surgical biopsy, FNA can provide information not only regarding a diagnosis but also information regarding staging and treatment as described above. US, CT, and endoscopic ultrasound are modalities that can be used to provide image guidance for FNA.

Suggested Reading

Atwell T, Charboneau JW, McGahan J, et al. Ultrasound-guided biopsy of abdomen and pelvis. In: Rumack CL, editor. Diagnostic ultrasound. Philadelphia: Mosby, Inc.; 2011. p. 613–38.

DeWitt J, Gress FJ, Levy M, et al. EUS-guided FNA aspiration of kidney masses: a multicenter US experience. Gastrointest Endosc. 2009;70:573–8.

DeWitt J, McGreevy K, Cummings O, et al. Initial experience with EUS-guided Tru-cut biopsy of benign liver disease. Gastrointest Endosc. 2009;69:535–42.

Khati NJ, Gorondenker J, Hill MC. Ultrasound-guided biopsies of the abdomen. Ultrasound Q. 2011;27:255–68.

Stelow EB, Debol SM, Stanley MW, et al. Sampling of the adrenal glands by endoscopic ultrasound-guided fine-needle aspiration. Diagn Cytopathol. 2005;33:26–30.

Chapter 2
On-Site Evaluation
and Specimen Preparation

Once FNA is performed, direct smears are prepared with one to two drops of fluid expressed from needle, typically two smears per needle pass. One smear is air dried and stained with Diff-Quik stain, and the second smear is wet-fixed in 95 % ethanol and later Papanicolaou stained. Residual material is rinsed from the needle into a balanced salt solution (e.g., Hanks) for ancillary studies or cell block (CB) preparation. Touch preparations of needle core biopsies (NCB) can also be performed if necessary for on-site evaluation. If the aspirator is working alone (i.e., no on-site evaluation), the specimen can be collected in a liquid-based cytology preservative solution for processing by ThinPrep (Cytyc Corporation, Marlborough, MA) or SurePath (BD, Franklin Lakes, NJ) techniques. The advantages of using liquid-based cytology include reduction in variability in smear quality, the ability to make multiple slide preparations for immunohistochemical staining and molecular studies, shorter screening time, and reduction in background debris, including tumor diathesis. The disadvantages include inability to perform real-time adequacy evaluation, submission of all material for Papanicolaou staining, and higher cost. NCBs are often performed in conjunction with FNA. Touch preparations of NCBs may also be performed for on-site evaluation, though not preferred because of the potential disruption/destruction of the NCB due to excess handling. On-site evaluation is

Y.S. Erozan and A. Tatsas, *Cytopathology of Liver, Biliary Tract, Kidney and Adrenal Gland*, Essentials in Cytopathology 18, DOI 10.1007/978-1-4899-7513-3_2, © Springer Science+Business Media New York 2015

extremely useful in specimen triage for flow cytometry studies, microbiology cultures, and for CB to perform immunocytochemistry or molecular studies. It is also useful to ensure target sampling for clinical research or trials.

Suggested Reading

Gill G. Cytopreparation—principals and practice, Essentials in cytopathology, vol. 12. New York: Springer; 2013.

Nasuti JF, Gupta PK, Baloch ZW. Diagnostic value and cost-effectiveness of on-site evaluation of fine-needle aspiration specimens: review of 5,688 cases. Diagn Cytopathol. 2002;27:1–4.

Schmidt RL, Witt BL, Lopez-Calderon LE, Layfield LJ. The influence of onsite evaluation on the adequacy rate of fine-needle aspiration cytology: a systematic review and meta-analysis. Am J Clin Pathol. 2013;139:300–8.

Chapter 3
Liver

Introduction

With the increasing use of imaging modalities to evaluate patients for primary diagnoses as well as to monitor patients with a history of malignancy, liver lesions are commonly identified. Autopsy studies indicate that in up to 50 % of patients, liver lesions may be detected and the vast majority of them are benign. Fine needle aspiration (FNA) of the liver is a useful tool to evaluate both solid and cystic lesions of the liver (Table 3.1). Benign and malignant lesions may be diagnosed by FNA, although the benign diagnoses may be difficult without a complementary needle core biopsy (NCB). Additionally, material obtained from FNA is well suited to microbiology cultures, flow cytometry studies, cytogenetic, and other molecular testing. FNA is not routinely indicated in the evaluation of hepatitis, cirrhosis, and metabolic diseases or for transplant monitoring.

Approach

Liver FNA is most often performed transabdominally under ultrasound or computed tomography (CT) guidance, typically by a radiologist. The advantages of ultrasound over CT guidance include real-time needle guidance, speed of procedure,

Y.S. Erozan and A. Tatsas, *Cytopathology of Liver, Biliary Tract, Kidney and Adrenal Gland*, Essentials in Cytopathology 18, DOI 10.1007/978-1-4899-7513-3_3, © Springer Science+Business Media New York 2015

TABLE 3.1.   Lesions that may be diagnosed on fine needle aspiration of liver.

- Fluid collections
    - Cysts
    - Abscesses
- Benign nodules/proliferations
    - Focal Nodular Hyperplasia
    - Liver cell adenoma
- Malignant neoplasms
    - Primary
    - Metastatic

excellent discrimination between solid and cystic lesions, lower cost of equipment, portability, and lack of radiation exposure. CT guidance offers better visualization of some lesions, particularly small ones.

MRI-guided procedures are possible, but require special equipment and are thus very expensive, and they rarely have any advantage in liver FNA. Transjugular biopsies performed using interventional radiology are rarely indicated (except for patients with impaired clotting, morbid obesity, or gross ascites) but may be attempted. "Blind" percutaneous liver biopsies (without image guidance) may be used in evaluation of diffuse liver abnormalities, but they are not typically used for targeting space-occupying lesions.

The newest technique is endoscopic ultrasound-guided FNA (EUS-FNA), which has a sensitivity of 82–94 % and specificity 90–100 % for space-occupying lesions. In these procedures, the liver is accessed via the stomach or small intestine. The left lobe of the liver is easily accessed, and the liver hilum, proximal right lobe, gallbladder, and perihilar lymph nodes can potentially be accessed. The technique is good for detecting and assessing a number of lesions for staging, and the diagnostic yield is higher for metastatic lesions than for primary HCC.

The approach to image-guided FNA is discussed in further detail in Chap. 1.

Sensitivity, Specificity, and Accuracy

The sensitivity of liver FNA ranges from 67 to 100 % and the specificity from 87 to 100 %. The overall accuracy is 80–95 %. The sensitivity and specificity for liver malignancy are 90 % and 100 %, and positive predictive value for malignancy approaches 100 %. Combined FNA and NCB has a higher sensitivity (85–100 %) compared to either FNA (62–100 %) or NCB alone (69–91 %).

Complications

The risk of complications is low, but the most commonly encountered ones include pain, hemorrhage, and infection. To control the associated pain, local anesthetic is typically provided with lidocaine, but the liver parenchyma cannot be anesthetized. Hemorrhage occurs in less than 1 % of patients. Intra-abdominal bleeding is the most severe potential complication, however transfusion is rarely required. The procedure is typically performed using sterile technique, and the rate of infection is less than 1 %. Prophylactic antimicrobials are not routinely given. The risk of tumor seeding due to the procedure is generally regarded as <0.01 %, though small series have reported a higher incidence of seeding in HCC (0.003–5.0 %). The risk of mortality is approximately 1 in 10,000–12,000.

Contraindications

Though generally a low-risk procedure, there are certain patients in whom liver FNA is contraindicated. Patients with severe bleeding disorders that cannot be corrected with therapy and those unable to remain still during the procedure or cooperate with positioning may be ineligible. Morbid obesity or massive ascites may impair the ability to perform transabdominal percutaneous liver biopsy, so the transjugular approach may be indicated. Some authorities suggest that aspiration of hepatocellular carcinoma carries a higher risk of bleeding and/or seeding, thus the procedure risks should be evaluated carefully in a borderline patient who is suspected to have HCC.

Complications of and contraindications to FNA are discussed in further detail in Chap. 1.

Normal Components of Liver

Hepatocytes

The predominant cell type in the liver is the hepatocyte, thus hepatocytes are frequently encountered in aspirates of non-neoplastic liver as well as admixed with neoplastic cells, both primary and metastatic. Aspirates of normal liver typically show a combination of loosely cohesive tissue fragments, small clusters of evenly spaced cells, or single cells. Fragments and small clusters have well-defined edges, and individual cells have well-defined cell borders. Single cells are round to polygonal, and cytoplasm is abundant and granular. The nuclear to cytoplasmic (n/c) ratio is low given the abundance of cytoplasm. Hepatocytes display a single, round nucleus which is centrally placed with smooth nuclear contours and may show a single small to variably prominent nucleolus. Occasional binucleation is encountered and is not indicative of dysplasia or neoplasia. Perinuclear accumulation of lipofuscin pigment is commonly encountered and is normal, increasing with patient age. Intranuclear inclusions are occasionally seen in normal hepatocytes, and their presence should not be taken as evidence of a hepatocellular neoplasm (Figs. 3.1, 3.2, and 3.3).

Key features:

- Tissue fragments, loosely cohesive small clusters or single cells
- Round to polygonal cells
- Well-defined cell borders

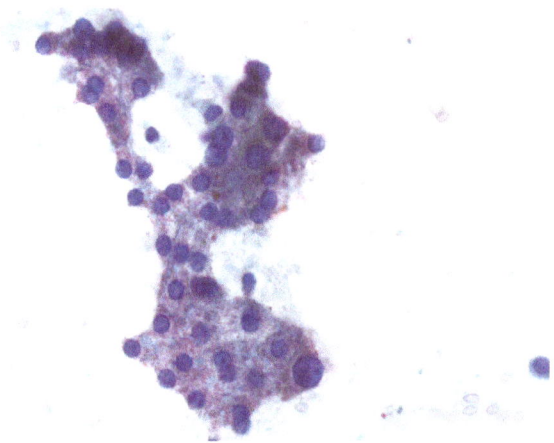

Fig. 3.1. Normal Hepatocytes: Hepatocytes have a polygonal shape with abundant coarsely granular cytoplasm and round nuclei with variably prominent nucleoli. The nuclear to cytoplasmic ratio is low due to the large volume of cytoplasm. (Papanicolaou stain, medium power)

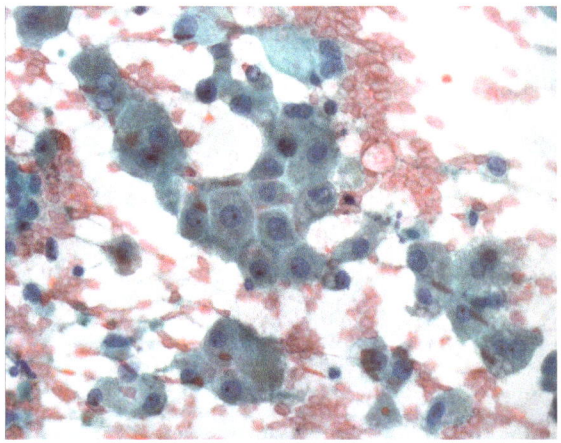

Fig. 3.2. Normal Hepatocytes: these hepatocytes are cohesive, forming a flat sheet of cells. They are polygonal and show abundant granular cytoplasm. Nuclei are round and centrally placed and have intermediate sized nucleoli. (Papanicolaou stain, high power)

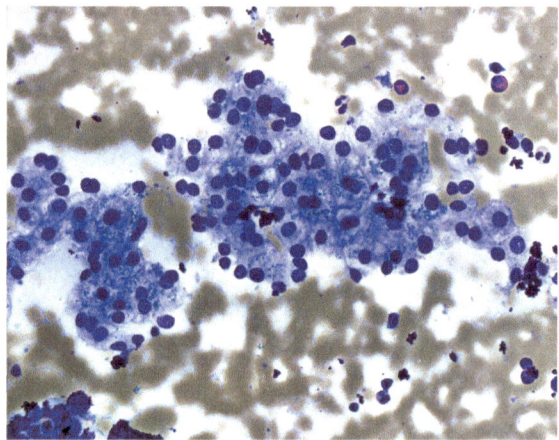

FIG. 3.3.   Normal Hepatocytes: A group of benign hepatocytes is shown demonstrating abundant granular cytoplasm and uniformly sized, round nuclei that are located in the center of the cell. There is some finely granular pigment present in the cytoplasm of some cells representing lipofuscin pigment. (Diff-Quik stain, medium power)

- Abundant granular cytoplasm
- Low nuclear to cytoplasmic ratio
- Centrally placed, round nucleus
- Smooth nuclear contours
- Single small to prominent nucleolus
- Perinuclear accumulation of lipofuscin pigment
- Scattered binucleation and intranuclear inclusions may be present

Biliary Ductal Epithelium

The second most common cell type encountered in aspirates of normal liver is biliary type epithelium, though it is usually present in much smaller quantity than hepatocytes. Ductal epithelium is typically present in flat, cohesive sheets of cells with evenly spaced nuclei showing no nuclear overlap or

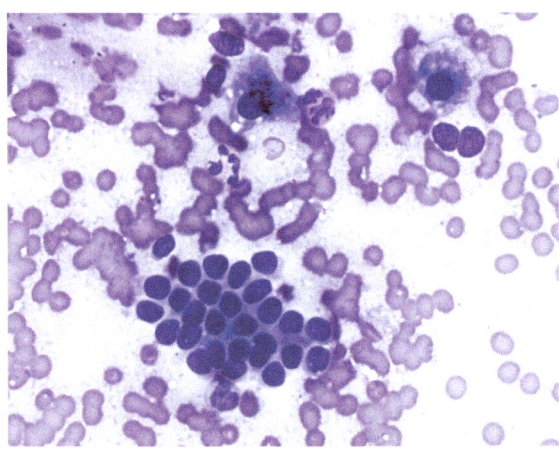

FIG. 3.4.   Normal Bile Duct: A cohesive fragment of epithelial cells is shown forming a flat sheet with evenly spaced nuclei showing minimal overlap. The nuclei are round to oval and show smooth nuclear contours. Biliary duct epithelium may present as flat sheets or acinar formations. (Diff-Quik stain, high power)

crowding. This "honeycomb" arrangement is similar to what is encountered in aspirates of pancreatic ductal epithelium. Small tubular or acinar structures are less commonly encountered (Fig. 3.4). The cells are overall smaller than hepatocytes, and the nuclear to cytoplasmic ratio is higher due to the presence of considerably less cytoplasm, though the nuclear sizes are similar in the two cell types. The cells are cuboidal to columnar in shape, nuclei are round to slightly oval and have absent to inconspicuous nucleoli.

Key features:

- Flat, cohesive sheets with "honeycomb" arrangement or small tubular or acinar structures
- Evenly spaced nuclei with no nuclear overlap or crowding
- Cuboidal to columnar cell shape
- Round to slightly oval nuclei
- Inconspicuous nucleoli
- Nuclear to cytoplasmic ratio higher than hepatocytes

Endothelial Cells

While endothelial cells are recognized as a key diagnostic feature in hepatocellular carcinoma, they are reported to be present in up to half of all aspirates of normal liver. They are not usually abundant in aspirates of benign liver and may not be noted. The cells are small and have spindle-shaped nuclei with smooth nuclear contours and a scant amount of delicate cytoplasm.

Kupffer Cells

These specialized macrophages assist in the degradation of hemoglobin to unconjugated bilirubin. They are cytomorphologically indistinguishable from normal macrophages and are thus not definitively identifiable on aspirate smears.

Contaminants

Mesothelial Cells

The main pitfall associated with the presence of mesothelial cells in liver aspirates is overinterpretation of these cells as an epithelial neoplasm. Recognition of this normal contaminant is generally straightforward on aspirate smears. Mesothelial cells appear most often as flat sheets or small fragments of uniformly sized cells which are evenly spaced and show no overlap. The nuclear to cytoplasmic ratio is typically low, and clear spaces between the cells ("windows") are a key defining feature. The nuclei are round to oval and may show occasional intranuclear grooves and small nucleoli (Fig. 3.5).

Key features:

- Flat sheets or small fragments of uniformly sized and spaced cells
- Nuclear to cytoplasmic ratio low
- Oval nuclei with occasional grooves and small nucleoli
- Characteristic clear spaces or "windows" between cells

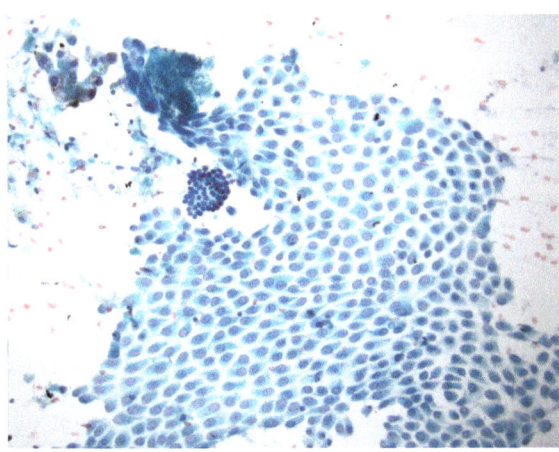

Fɪɢ. 3.5.   Normal Mesothelial cells: A large flat sheet of mesothelial cells is present and shows clear spaces ("windows") between evenly spaced cells. The nuclei are round with evenly dispersed nuclei and occasional grooves. A small group of hepatocytes is present in the *upper left corner*, and a group of bile duct epithelium is present at 10 o'clock, just to the *upper left of center*. (Papanicolaou stain, medium power)

Gastric Wall

Fragments of gastric epithelium may be aspirated in transabdominal aspirates targeting the left hepatic lobe. The epithelium is columnar and may display mucinous features. The overall appearance should be bland and nuclei should be small and well organized.

Pulmonary/Respiratory Epithelium

Just as hepatic tissue may be acquired unintentionally in sampling of the right lower lung, it is possible to encounter pulmonary or respiratory epithelium in aspirates targeting the hepatic dome. The epithelium may show cilia, or could show features of benign pneumocytes and alveolar macrophages. Knowledge of the precise lesion location may help confirm this contamination.

Skeletal Muscle and Skin

Skin may contaminate an aspirate of the liver if it is acquired transabdominally. Fragments of skin are typically cohesive and show organized epithelium with little nuclear overlap. Skeletal muscle may be encountered if the diaphragm is aspirated.

Pigments (Table 3.2)

Lipofuscin

This normal "wear and tear" pigment is a result of debris produced from the breakdown of intracellular lysosomes. It is a normal component of the hepatocyte and accumulates with aging. It is found in a perinuclear location and is finely granular. Lipofuscin is golden-brown in color on Papanicolaou stain, dark green-brown on Diff-Quik and is not refractile. The absence of lipofuscin in all of the hepatocytes in an aspirated sample may raise the suspicion for a neoplastic process.

TABLE 3.2.   Pigments encountered in liver aspirates.

Pigments	Lipofuscin	Bile	Hemosiderin	Melanin
Location	Perinuclear	Cytoplasmic, extracellular	Cytoplasmic, macrophages	Cytoplasmic, macrophages
Color on Papanicolaou stain	Golden-brown	Green to green-brown	Golden-brown	Brown
Color on Diff-Quik	Dark green-brown	Dark green to black	Dark blue	Dark blue to black
Size/texture	Fine	Amorphous/ globular	Coarse	Finely granular
Refractile	No	No	Yes	No
Context	Normal, aging	Hepatitis, Cholestasis, HCC	Hemochromatosis, transfusions	Melanoma

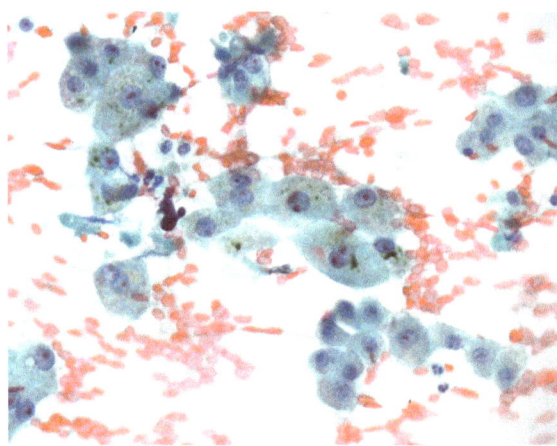

Fig. 3.6.   Hepatocytes, benign with bile: These hepatocytes show abundant granular cytoplasm with round nuclei, some showing prominent nucleoli. Globular *green* to *brown* pigment is present in many cells, most notable in the center of the image. Bile stasis may result from a number of neoplastic and nonneoplastic conditions. (Papanicolaou stain, high power)

Bile

Bile is produced in the hepatocytes and stored in the gallbladder. Increased accumulation of bile occurs in a number of nonneoplastic and neoplastic settings in the liver. The presence of bile in a clearly malignant process strongly supports hepatocellular origin. Bile may be variable in color, texture, and density, but is generally coarse, irregular, and amorphous. It is not refractile and stains green to green-brown on Papanicolaou stain and dark green to black on Diff-Quik (Fig. 3.6).

Hemosiderin

Iron pigment, or hemosiderin, is encountered in hepatocytes, bile duct epithelial cells, and Kupffer cells. It is a coarse pigment, appearing golden-brown on Papanicolaou stain, but dark blue to black on Diff-Quik stain. It is refractile, in contrast to bile and lipofuscin pigments. Malignant hepato-cytes lose ability to retain iron, so a Prussian blue iron stain may be helpful to confirm a diagnosis of HCC (negative stain-ing), though it is not routinely used for diagnosis of HCC.

Melanin

Though not a normal component of liver aspirates, melanin may be present in cases of metastatic melanoma. The neo-plastic cells of melanoma can show some morphologic over-lap with hepatocytes, including prominent nucleoli and intranuclear inclusions. Melanin pigment is finely granular and brown on Papanicolaou stain and dark blue to black on Diff-Quik.

Nonneoplastic Processes and Benign Nodules

Infections

Hydatid Cysts

Though most commonly seen in South America, Australia, New Zealand, and Mediterranean countries, hydatid cysts are occasionally encountered in the United States. Overall, they are the most common cause of hepatic cysts worldwide. They are caused by dog tapeworm, *Echinococcus granulosus*, most commonly, or *Echinococcus multilocularis*. These cysts may remain asymptomatic until they become very large and can be fatal if left untreated. The cysts are typically not aspirated if suspected clinically as leakage of the contents may result in anaphylactic shock, though the actual likelihood of this is debated.

Radiographically, hydatid cysts typically present as a soli-tary lesion. Cyst wall calcification may be evident on imaging, and septae may be detected within the cyst. Grossly, they are usually unilocular. A peripheral rim of calcification is seen in 25 % of cases. On histologic sections, a laminated cyst wall is

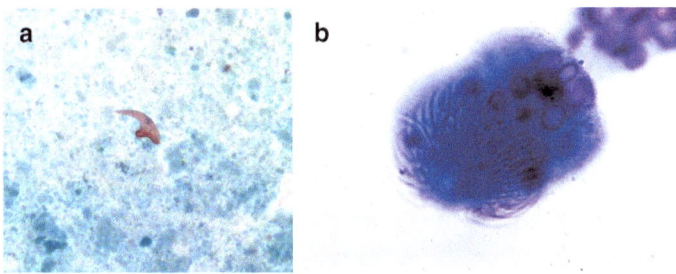

Fig. 3.7.   Hydatid cyst: (**a**) A hooklet from an echinococcal cyst is shown in the *center* of the field with a "whale's tooth" shape. The background shows abundant granular, necrotic debris. (Papanicolaou stain, medium power). (**b**) A scolex from echinococcal cyst. (Diff-Quik stain, high power)

seen, often with acellular debris within the cyst. The wall of the cyst is surrounded by mixed acute and chronic inflammation with abundant eosinophils. Aspiration yields clear, colorless cyst fluid. Granular inflammatory debris is abundant with the presence of hooklets or scolices confirming the diagnosis. Hooklets are often degenerated, but are 20–40 μm in size, have a "shark's tooth" shape, and are refractile (Fig. 3.7a). They are positive with acid-fast stains. Occasionally a large scolex, or worm head, composed of multiple hooklets is seen, but these may degenerate and be difficult to detect (Fig. 3.7b).

Key features:
Granular inflammatory debris

- Hooklets
    - Often degenerated
    - Shark's tooth shape
    - Acid fast positive

- Occasional scolices

Differential diagnosis:
The differential diagnosis includes other parasitic cysts, including those caused by *Entamoeba*, *Clonorchis*, or *Schistosoma* species. In addition, other typically unilocular

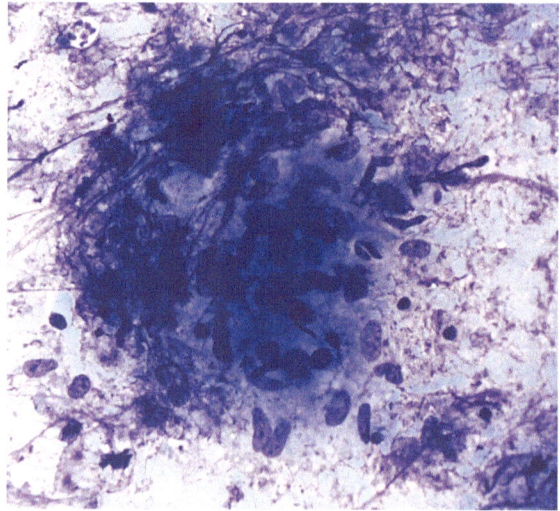

FIG. 3.8.   Granuloma: This is a loose aggregation of histiocytes
showing abundant cytoplasm and oval to comma-shaped nuclei.
There are scattered admixed small lymphocytes. The origin of the
granulomatous inflammation cannot be determined from the aspirate smear in this case. (Diff-Quik stain, medium power)

cysts which may occur in the liver include simple cyst (lined
by biliary, ciliated, or squamous epithelium), ciliated foregut
cyst, and pseudocyst.

Granulomatous Inflammation

In general, granulomatous inflammation is seen in a number
of conditions including sarcoidosis, infection, drug reaction,
primary biliary cirrhosis, and in the setting of some neoplasms (particularly hematopoietic). A specific etiology is not
usually evident on cytopathologic material unless organisms
are identified on aspirate smears. Cytopathologically, clusters
of epithelioid histiocytes are seen admixed with variable
numbers of multinucleated giant cells (Figs. 3.8 and 3.9).
If granulomatous inflammation is seen on on-site evaluation,

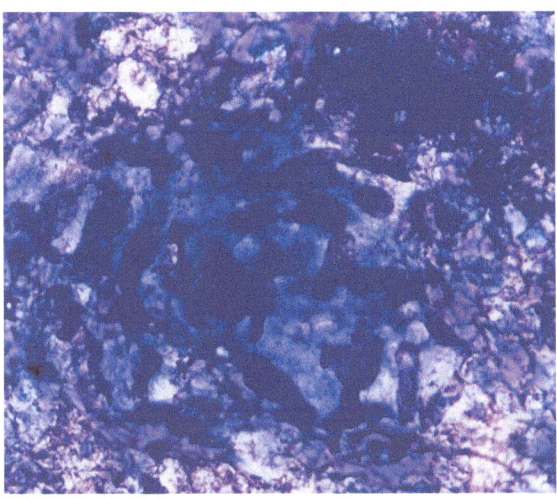

Fɪɢ. 3.9.   Granuloma: A cluster of histiocytes is shown with abundant cytoplasm, ill-defined cell borders, and oval to comma-shaped nuclei. Small lymphocytes are embedded in the cluster consistent with a granuloma. (Diff-Quik stain, high power)

aspirates of the lesion should be sent for culture. If an accompanying CB or NCB is available, special stains for organisms can be performed, though culture is preferable.

Pyogenic Abscess

Pyogenic abscesses are most often the result of bacterial infection, usually a polymicrobial infection. *Escherichia coli* is the most common infectious agent isolated from pyogenic abscesses. Radiographically, these lesions may show a "double-target sign" on CT. Aspirate smears show acute inflammation and cellular debris. Collection of material for bacterial, fungal, and acid fast cultures is essential.

Extramedullary Hematopoiesis

Although normally present in infants, extramedullary hematopoiesis (EMH) is an abnormal finding in adults and older children. It is seen in adults as a result of bone marrow failure. Aspirates are composed of all of the elements normally present in a bone marrow aspirate including erythroid, myeloid, and lymphoid cells at various stages of maturation (Figs. 3.10 and 3.11). The presence of megakaryocytes is the most striking feature and may be mistaken for neoplasm such as a high grade sarcoma or carcinoma if EMH is not considered (Fig. 3.12). The presence of a mixed hematopoietic population in the background should raise the possibility of EMH.

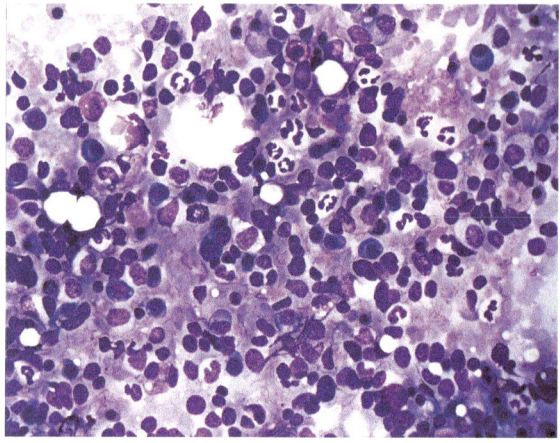

FIG. 3.10.   Extramedullary hematopoiesis: This field shows a mixture of immature hematopoietic cells including erythroid, myeloid, and lymphoid precursors. Mature neutrophils and a few plasma cells are also admixed. (Diff-Quik stain, high power)

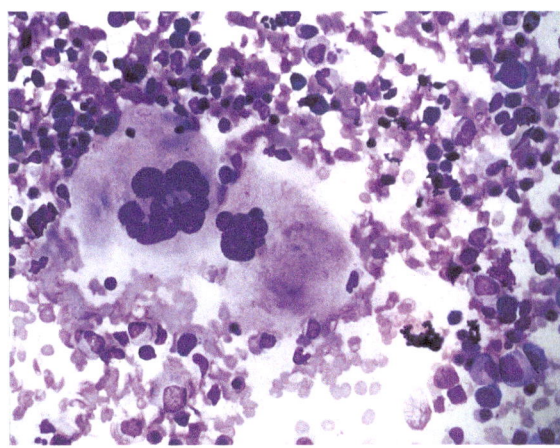

FIG. 3.11. Extramedullary hematopoiesis: Two megakaryocytes are shown in the *center/left* of the field surrounded by a mixed population of immature hematopoietic cells. Scattered megakaryocytes or bare megakaryocyte nuclei may be misinterpreted as a malignant neoplasm if EMH is not considered. (Diff-Quik stain, high power)

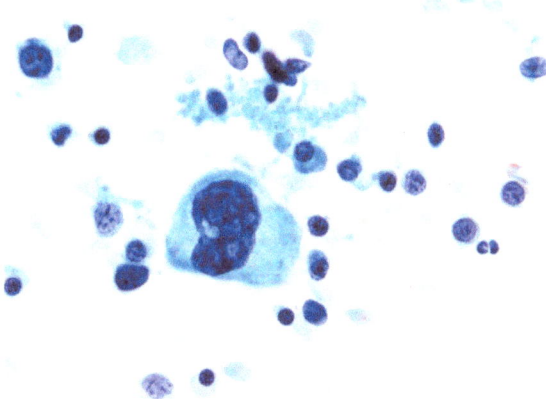

FIG. 3.12. Extramedullary hematopoiesis: A megakaryocyte is shown at the *center* of the screen surrounded by immature hematopoietic cells. Many of the smaller cells in the background are more difficult to distinguish from mature lymphocytes on Papanicolaou as opposed to Diff-Quik preparations. (Papanicolaou stain, high power)

Hemangioma

Hepatic hemangiomas are very common lesions, found in up to 20 % of the general population. They have a female predominance and typically range from 1 to 10 cm in size. Small lesions are usually asymptomatic, but large ones may be symptomatic causing abdominal pain, anorexia, or nausea. There is a low risk of rupture, but these lesions may enlarge during pregnancy or during oral contraceptive use. They are most often solitary and have a characteristic radiographic appearance, thus they are not usually aspirated. If aspirated, cytopathologic features include abundant blood, scant pauci-cellular fibrous tissue, and, rarely, small groups of endothelial cells having spindle-shaped nuclei with tapered ends forming a swirling or streaming pattern (Figs. 3.13 and 3.14). CB or NCB can be quite useful if even a small amount of the lesion is obtained. The diagnosis should be considered in samples deemed "inadequate."

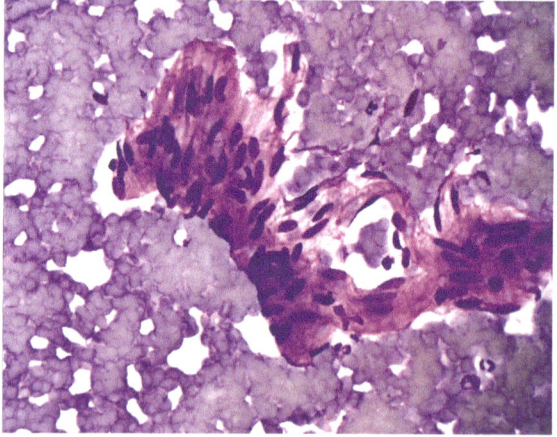

Fig. 3.13.   Hemangioma: A small fragment of cohesive spindle cells is shown and shows a suggestion of lumen formation. Aspirates of hemangiomas are typically sparsely cellular and show a bloody background. (Diff-Quik stain, high power)

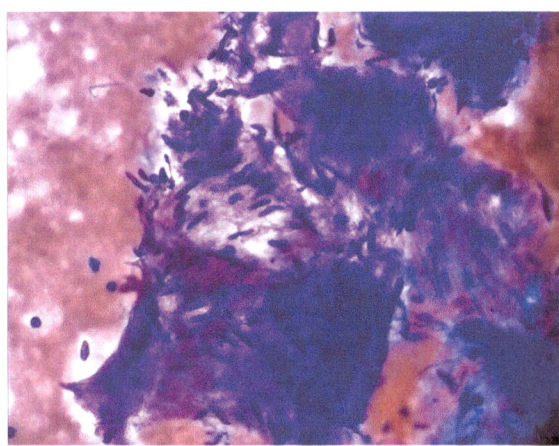

Fɪɢ. 3.14. Hemangioma: Fibrous tissue with embedded bland spindle cells is present in a background of blood. A low grade spindle cell neoplasm would be included in the differential diagnosis. Even a small NCB can be very helpful in making the diagnosis in this situation. (Diff-Quik stain, high power)

Key features:

- Very scant cellularity
- Bloody background
- Scant fibrous stroma
- Few spindled endothelial cells

Differential diagnosis:

The differential diagnosis includes unsampled neoplasm as the lesion may appear insufficient for diagnosis. If spindle cells are encountered, one should consider spindle cell neoplasms such as angiosarcoma, epithelioid hemangioendothelioma, metastatic gastrointestinal stromal tumor (GIST), or leiomyosarcoma. The degree of pleomorphism is typically much greater in the spindle cell neoplasms, and CB or NCB may be quite useful in distinguishing these lesions.

Cirrhosis

Over half of cases of cirrhosis in the United States are caused
by alcoholic liver disease. Other common causes of cirrhosis
include viral hepatitis, hemochromatosis, nonalcoholic steato-
hepatitis, and autoimmune diseases. FNA is not useful to
grade cirrhosis, but cirrhotic liver may be sampled as part of a
workup for a solid mass, thus knowledge of the cytopathologic
features is essential. Cirrhosis is characterized histologically
by diffuse fibrous bands separating nodules of hepatocytes
that show varying degrees of atypia including increased
nuclear size and prominent nucleoli (Fig. 3.15). Masson trichrome stain highlights the fibrosis (Fig. 3.16). Similarly, morphologic features range from normal appearing to variably
atypical hepatocytes. Focal marked anisocytosis may be

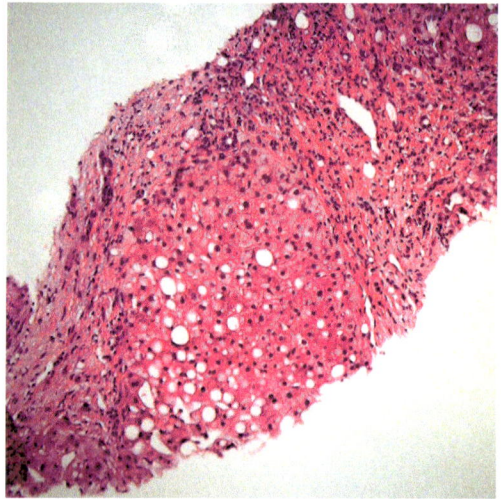

FIG. 3.15.   Cirrhosis: A nodule of hepatocytes surrounded by dense
fibrous bands is shown. The hepatocytes show steatosis and some
nuclear enlargement. These features of mild atypia are also seen in
aspirate smears from cirrhotic livers. (Core biopsy. H&E stain,
medium power)

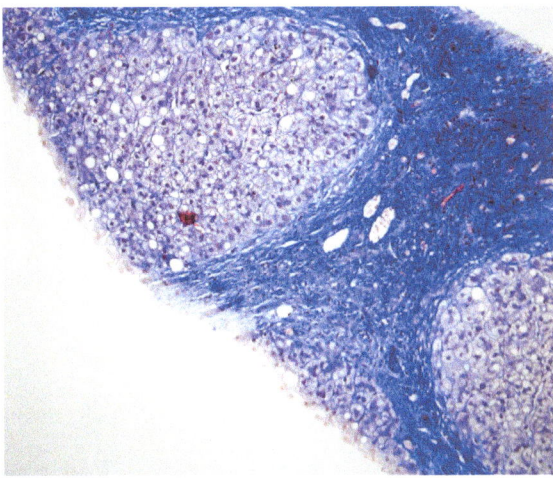

Fig. 3.16.   Cirrhosis: This Masson trichrome stain highlights the dense fibrous tissue surrounding nodules of hepatocytes. Steatosis and nuclear atypia including enlargement can be seen. (Core biopsy, Masson trichrome stain, medium power)

present, and binucleation is not uncommon. The nuclear to cytoplasmic ratio may be normal to slightly increased. Prominent nucleoli and intranuclear inclusions are commonly seen. Typically there is some fibrous tissue aspirated and admixed with hepatocytes, and there is usually abundant bile duct epithelium present, in contrast to hepatic adenomas and hepatocellular carcinoma (Figs. 3.17, 3.18, and 3.19).

Key features:

- Normal to variably atypical hepatocytes
- Focal marked anisocytosis
- Binucleation
- Prominent nucleoli
- Intranuclear inclusions
- Normal to slightly increased n/c ratio
- Scant to moderate fibrous tissue
- Abundant bile duct epithelium

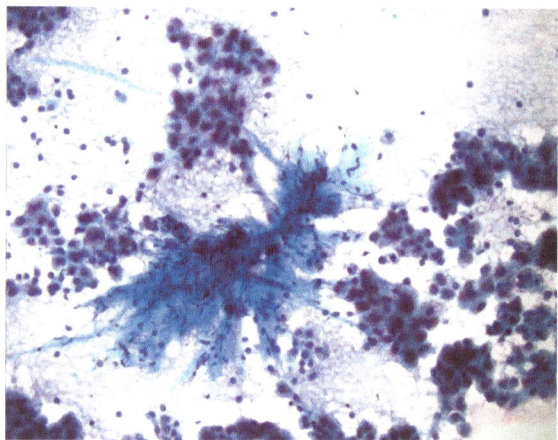

FIG. 3.17.   Cirrhosis: A fragment of dense fibrous tissue is shown in the *center* of the field surrounded by small fragments of hepatocytes. The hepatocytes show scattered nuclear enlargement and occasional binucleation. There are very few single cells present. (Papanicolaou stain, medium power)

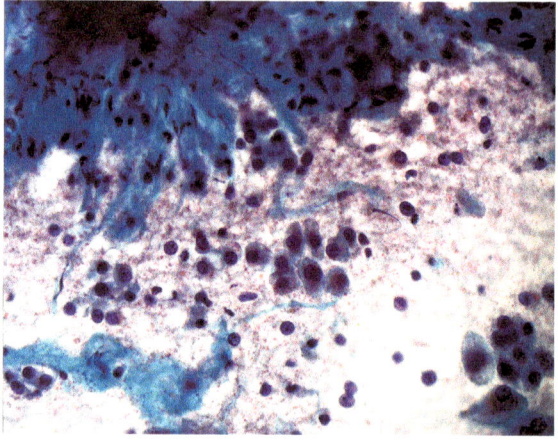

FIG. 3.18.   Cirrhosis: Single hepatocytes with mild nuclear enlargement and scattered binucleation are shown adjacent to a fragment of dense fibrous tissue. (Papanicolaou stain, high power)

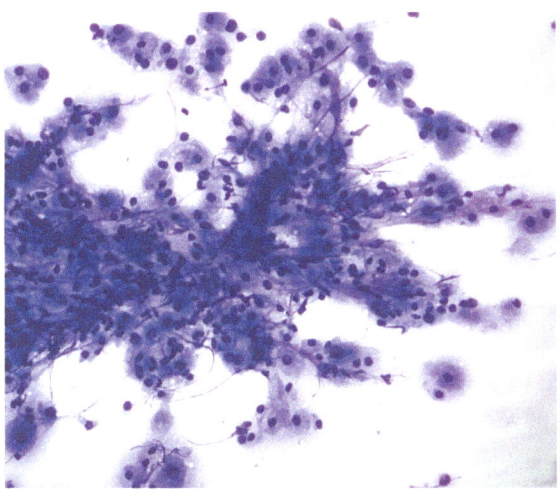

FIG. 3.19.   Cirrhosis: This fragment shows hepatocytes with mild nuclear atypia intimately admixed with dense fibrous tissue. There is no vascular pattern or marked atypia to suggest a hepatocellular neoplasm. (Diff-Quik stain, high power)

Regenerative or Dysplastic Nodules

Macroregenerative Nodules

Macroregenerative nodules are nodules 1 cm or larger in a background of cirrhosis. They are also known as large regencrative nodules or adenomatous hyperplasia. Histologically they resemble cirrhotic nodules with an intact reticulin framework and cell plates one to two cells thick. Cytopathologically they show a uniform population of hepatocytes with some nuclear atypia. Whole cellular and nuclear enlargements are common, but the nuclear to cytoplasmic ratio is maintained (approximately 1:3). The nuclei show smooth nuclear membranes. It is also possible to encounter Mallory bodies, bile stasis, iron deposition, or focal fatty change depending on the underlying etiology of cirrhosis.

The differential diagnosis includes focal nodular hyperplasia and well-differentiated hepatocellular carcinoma, though distinction is not possible on cytology.

Dysplastic Nodules

Dysplastic nodules also occur in a background of cirrhotic liver and may display either "large cell" or "small cell" change. Large cell change morphologically consists of cellular enlargement, nuclear pleomorphism, and multinucleation, and it is controversial as to whether it is a direct precursor lesion to HCC. Small cell change, on the other hand, is considered premalignant and is present in up to 50 % of cirrhotic liver explants. Morphologically, hepatocytes show overall decreased cytoplasmic volume, cytoplasmic basophilia, mild nuclear pleomorphism, and hyperchromasia. There is an increased nuclear to cytoplasmic ratio given the reduction in cytoplasmic volume. These nodules show focal loss of reticulin framework, which must be evaluated on tissue sections. The differential diagnosis includes a well-differentiated HCC, and tissue evidence of stromal invasion is needed to distinguish these two.

Focal Nodular Hyperplasia (FNH)

This typically asymptomatic condition is often discovered incidentally in patients undergoing imaging for an unrelated complaint. It is more common in women, particularly in the age range of 20–40 years. Formation of FNH is not associated with oral contraceptive use, however use may result in enlargement and increase in vascularity. There is no association with hemoperitoneum. They are usually less than 3 cm in size and arise in noncirrhotic livers. This condition is either treated with local or segmental liver resection or followed radiographically (small lesions). Radiographically, a characteristic central stellate scar is usually evident, and tissue diagnosis is often not necessary. Histologically these

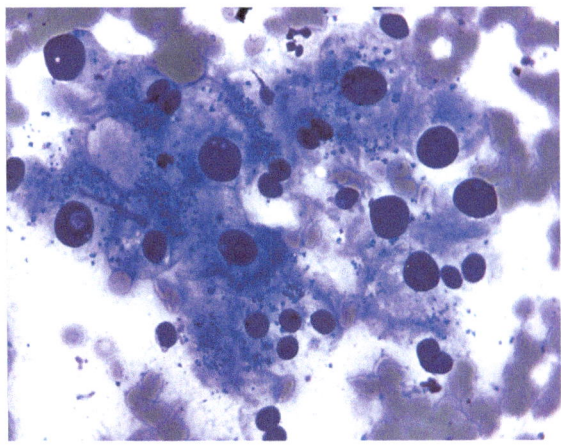

FIG. 3.20.   Focal nodular hyperplasia: These hepatocytes show anisonucleosis with some marked nuclear enlargement. The nuclei are
still round and centrally placed in the cells. (Diff-Quik stain, high
power)

lesion resemble "focal cirrhosis," that is nodules of bland
hepatocytes surrounded by bands of fibrosis with bile duct
proliferation at the periphery of the nodule. No portal
tracts or central veins are present within the lesion.
Cytopathologically, normal to hyperplastic hepatocytes may
show binucleation and may be present as two cell thick
groups. Otherwise the hepatocytes show normal morphology
and nuclear to cytoplasmic ratio. Fatty change may be seen,
and numerous bile ducts are present, some forming long
tubules. Fibrous tissue is typically sparse on aspirate smears.
In contrast to HCC, there is no endothelial proliferation and
the reticulin framework is intact (Figs. 3.20 and 3.21).

Differential diagnosis:
Correlation with radiographic findings to rule out cirrhosis
or normal liver is essential to the diagnosis. Based on morphology alone, the differential includes well-differentiated
HCC, which typically occurs in a cirrhotic liver and shows
increased thickness of cell plates (>2 cells), which can be

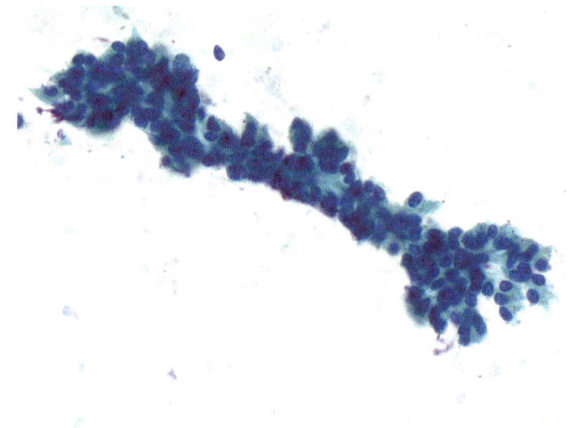

Fig. 3.21.   Focal nodular hyperplasia: This long tubular structure is a bile duct. The nuclei are small and uniformly sized with smooth nuclear contours. Abundant bile duct epithelium, some forming large tubular structures are common in FNH. (Papanicolaou stain, high power)

confirmed with reticulin. A hepatic adenoma is also in the differential, but the two cannot be reliably distinguished based on cytology alone.

Hepatic (Liver Cell) Adenoma

Hepatic adenomas (HAs) are much more common in women than men and are seen most often in patients under 30 years of age. They are strongly associated with oral contraceptive use (>5 years). They are often symptomatic, and abdominal pain is common, particularly with intratumoral hemorrhage. Spontaneous rupture and hemoperitoneum occur in 10 % of cases, especially during menstruation, pregnancy, or postpartum. Radiologically, they are seen to arise in noncirrhotic livers and are most often solitary. They are homogeneous lesions with no central scar, and hemorrhage within the lesion suggests adenoma. On histologic sections, HAs are well-defined neoplasms consisting of hepatocytes with normal (nonthickened) hepatic plates (one to two cells thick). They lack portal triads and central veins, and steatosis is common. FNAs are hypercellular and show a monotonous population of normal hepatocytes. Hepatocytes occur singly and in cords two cells thick and show minimal nuclear atypia with normal nuclear to cytoplasmic ratio. Bile ducts should be absent, though the diagnosis of HA is not completely excluded by the presence of bile ducts, as they may be sampled from surrounding normal liver.

Differential diagnosis:
Just as in FNH, it is essential that one correlate the cytomorphology with radiographic findings to rule out cirrhosis or normal liver. The differential includes a well-differentiated HCC and immunostains, including CD34, can be helpful in making the distinction. FNH is also in the differential, but the two cannot be distinguished reliably on FNA.

Bile Duct Adenoma

These are small (<2 cm) lesions, commonly encountered during intra-abdominal surgery due to their subcapsular location. They are well circumscribed and histologically composed of a bland bile duct proliferation and fibrosis. They are not often aspirated, but when they are, they show abundant bile duct epithelium in flat sheet and scant hepatocytes.

Differential diagnosis:
The differential diagnosis includes von Meyenburg complex, which typically show multiple lesions and have intraluminal bile present. Well-differentiated cholangiocarcinoma or metastatic adenocarcinoma may be considered, though bile duct adenoma should not have nuclear atypia. Radiographic and clinical correlation is also important.

Angiomyolipoma

Angiomyolipoma (AML) is a rare primary liver tumor. It occurs in male and female patients with similar incidence, and is most common in patients 30–40 years of age. Most are asymptomatic. They display similar histologic and cytomorphologic findings to AML in kidney, including a combination of fat, smooth muscle and blood vessels. The fat component is more often scant or absent in liver versus kidney. Spindle cell lesions are considered in the differential. The main pitfall is the epithelioid variant, which may be misinterpreted as carcinoma, particularly HCC, due to cells with abundant eosinophilic cytoplasm and formation of trabeculae. The distinction is based on absence of cirrhosis in background liver and lack of nucleoli, bile, and fatty change within tumor cells. Immunoreactivity for HMB-45 and SMA, along with negativity for cytokeratin, confirms the diagnosis of AML.

Hepatobiliary Cystadenoma

This rare lesion is seen predominantly in middle-aged women and is associated with cystadenomas of the pancreas and ovary. Patients may present with abdominal pain. They have a thick septated wall and histologically are lined by a single layer of mucinous epithelial cells (flat, cuboidal, or columnar). The stroma in women shows ovarian morphology and is positive for ER and PR. Importantly, up to 25 % undergo malignant transformation to cystadenocarcinoma, so surgical resection is indicated. On cytology smears, they are composed of benign-appearing ductal epithelium with mucinous cells and goblet cells having bland, uniformly sized nuclei without nucleoli. There is often extracellular mucin. Ovarian stroma is not typically aspirated, and there should be absent or very few hepatocytes (from needle pickup only). Hepatobiliary cystadenocarcinoma is the main differential diagnostic consideration and shows atypical glandular epithelium. Surgical resection may be required to distinguish the two.

Primary Hepatic Malignant Neoplasms

Improvements in dynamic imaging techniques, such as contrast-enhanced ultrasound and dynamic magnetic resonance imaging (MR), have greatly increased the accuracy of diagnosis of hepatocellular carcinoma in patients with cirrhosis, obviating the need for tissue confirmation in many cases with the classic presentation of HCC. Thus, the nodules that cytopathologists are asked to evaluate are smaller (less than 2 cm) and show fewer of the characteristic clinical and radiographic features of HCC than hepatic nodules evaluated in the past.

Cholangiocarcinoma is the second most common primary liver malignancy, though far less common than HCC. It should be distinguished from metastatic carcinomas, which are discussed in detail later in this chapter.

Hepatocellular Carcinoma (HCC)

Though more rare in the United States, HCC is the sixth most common malignancy and third leading cause of cancer deaths worldwide. It is most common in Asia and sub-Saharan Africa due to endemic hepatitis B and aflatoxin B1. Incidence is rising in the West, however, as a consequence of increased Hepatitis C infection and nonalcoholic fatty liver disease. Risk factors for HCC include cirrhosis as 90–95 % of HCCs arise in a cirrhotic liver and the incidence of HCC is 1–6 % in cirrhotic patients. Particular associations include alcohol abuse, Hepatitis B and C viral infection, metabolic liver disease, environmental carcinogens, smoking, and hereditary hemochromatosis. It is important to realize, though, that in the United States metastases are 20–40 times more common in noncirrhotic livers. Primary hepatic lesions, primarily HCC, do outnumber metastases in the cirrhotic liver by three to one. Over 80 % of masses larger than 2 cm in a cirrhotic liver are HCC and 75 % of masses <2 cm in a cirrhotic liver are HCC. Overall the tumor has a very poor prognosis. FNA has a high sensitivity for the diagnosis of HCC, but in those with

a negative (false) diagnosis, repeat FNA only returns a definitive diagnosis in approximately one-third due to sampling of
small lesions or vast necrotic areas in large tumors.

Clinical Features, Signs, and Symptoms

Clinically, patients with HCC most often have underlying cirrhosis. Symptoms include new abdominal pain, recent hepatomegaly, hemoperitoneum, persistent fever, weight loss, a
sudden increase in alkaline phosphatase, increased AST to
ALT ratio, and persistent leukocytosis. Serum alpha-
fetoprotein (AFP) is typically elevated, though 20 % of all
HCCs produce no AFP. An AFP greater than 400 ng/mL suggests HCC, but 30 % of patients with HCC smaller than 2 cm
have normal AFP. The presence of these signs and symptoms,
particularly in a cirrhotic patient, should prompt consideration of a diagnosis of HCC.

Radiographic Features

HCC most often presents as a single large mass but may have
multiple smaller nodules. Rarely, diffuse liver enlargement is
present. Dynamic imaging modalities (US and MR) have
very high accuracy, sensitivity, and specificity (99.6, 100, and
98.9 %) for HCC. In fact, no tissue confirmation is required
if there is intense enhancement in the arterial phase with
contrast washout in the delayed venous phase on one
dynamic imaging modality. Nodules between 1 and 2 cm in
cirrhotic livers require concurrence of two imaging modalities,
otherwise tissue confirmation is required. Some suggest an
every 3-month surveillance approach in lesions <1 cm, but
68 % of these nodules detected in cirrhotic livers are HCC.

Histology

On tissue sections, HCC shows a loss of normal hepatic
and sinusoidal architecture, including cell plates greater than
two hepatocytes thick, absent portal triads and central veins,

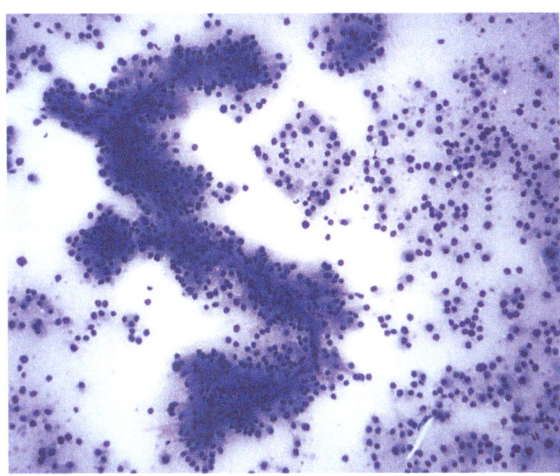

FIG. 3.22.   Hepatocellular Carcinoma: A large tissue fragment is present showing a blood vessel transgressing the entire length of the fragment. Numerous single hepatocytes are present in the background. There is mild nuclear enlargement and these findings are characteristic of a well-differentiated HCC. (Diff-Quik stain, low power)

and hepatocyte atypia, which increases with increasing grade. The architecture may be trabecular (most common), acinar, or solid.

Cytomorphology, HCC, General

In general, FNA of HCC yields a hypercellular aspirate composed of cellular fragments and single cells (Fig. 3.22), often with numerous bare nuclei in the background. "Wide" trabecular architecture (many cell layers thick) is present within tissue fragments. The vascular pattern seen on aspirate smears is key to the diagnosis of HCC. The presence of nests of tumor enveloped by endothelium at the periphery (endothelial wrapping) is virtually pathognomonic and very helpful when present (Figs. 3.23, 3.24, and 3.25). Though slightly less specific, the presence of a "transgressing or arborizing"

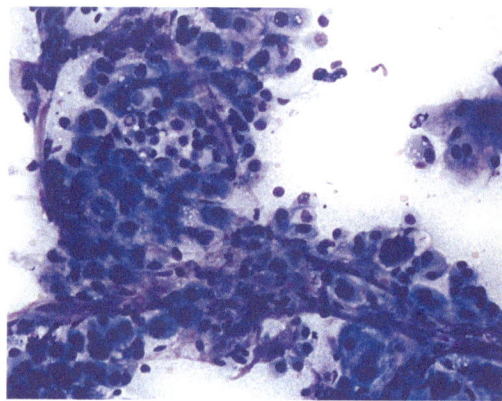

FIG. 3.23. Hepatocellular Carcinoma, endothelial wrapping: Endothelial cells are shown both wrapping around a group of malignant hepatocytes (*upper left*) and transgressing the center of the tissue fragment (*bottom*). Hepatocytes show binucleation, nuclear enlargement, and scattered intranuclear inclusions (10 o'clock). (Diff-Quik stain, medium power)

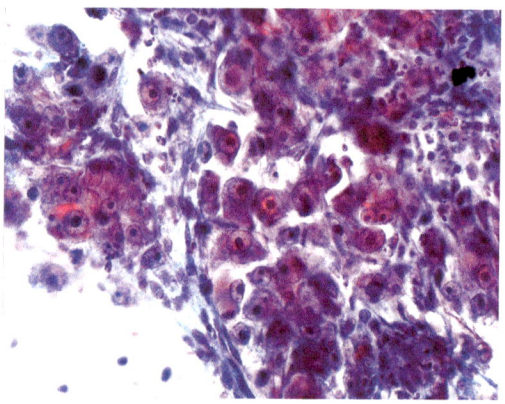

FIG. 3.24.   Hepatocellular Carcinoma, endothelial wrapping: On high magnification, the delicate spindle-shaped endothelial cells can be seen wrapping around a group of neoplastic hepatocytes. The hepatocytes show marked nuclear atypia including nuclear enlargement, binucleation, and macronucleoli. (Papanicolaou stain, high power)

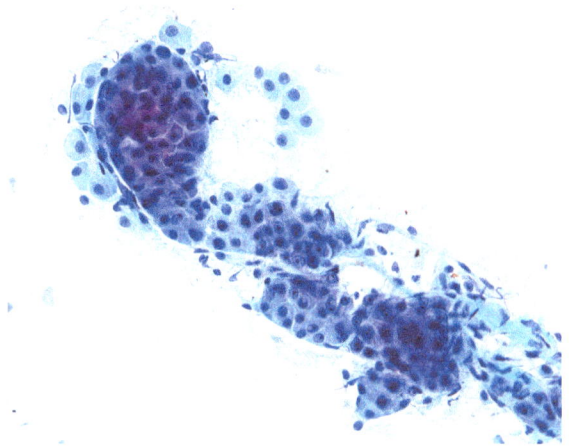

FIG. 3.25.   Hepatocellular Carcinoma: Few scattered small spindle cells are seen at the periphery of these fragments of HCC. In some cases of HCC, the endothelial cells are scarce, but typically can be found if the cells are carefully examined. (Papanicolaou stain, medium power)

vascular pattern showing a complex network of small vessels traversing loosely cohesive sheets of hepatocytes is very characteristic of HCC (Figs. 3.26 and 3.27). The tumor cells are relatively monomorphous, particularly in well- and moderately differentiated HCC. Cells are variably sized, and there are polygonal cells with well-defined cell borders and abundant granular cytoplasm. Nucleoli are often prominent, and numerous intranuclear inclusions may be seen, though these are not specific for HCC and can be seen in normal or reactive hepatocytes. The nuclear to cytoplasmic ratio increases with grade (Figs. 3.28, 3.29, and 3.30). Bile ducts are absent from the background. Bile pigment is highly specific for HCC versus metastatic carcinoma. Additional features include possible intracytoplasmic fat, glycogen (PAS +), and eosinophilic cytoplasmic inclusions resembling Mallory hyaline. Specific features for well-, moderately, and poorly differentiated HCC are enumerated below.

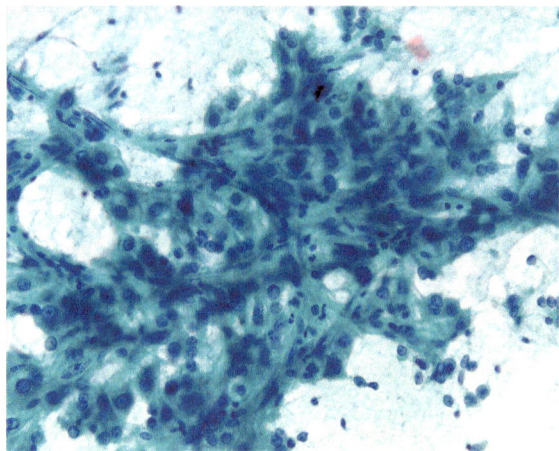

FIG. 3.26.   Hepatocellular Carcinoma, transgressing blood vessels: This large fragment of malignant hepatocytes shows vessels traversing the length of the fragment in many directions. A monotonous population of hepatocytes surrounds the spindled endothelial cells. (Papanicolaou stain, high power)

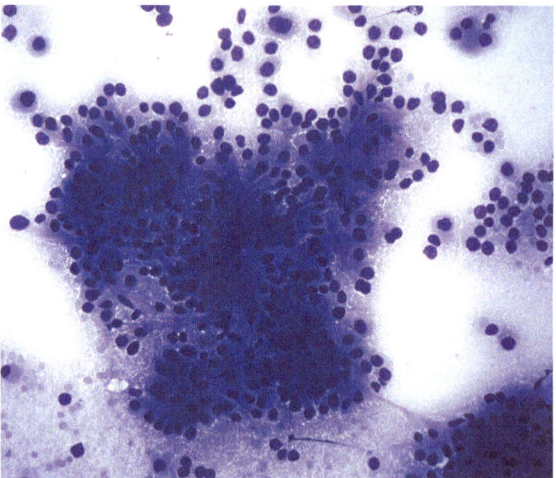

FIG. 3.27.   Hepatocellular Carcinoma: This fragment shows transgressing small blood vessels admixed with hepatocytes. The hepatocytes are generally bland, but show some nuclear enlargement. (Diff-Quik stain, medium power)

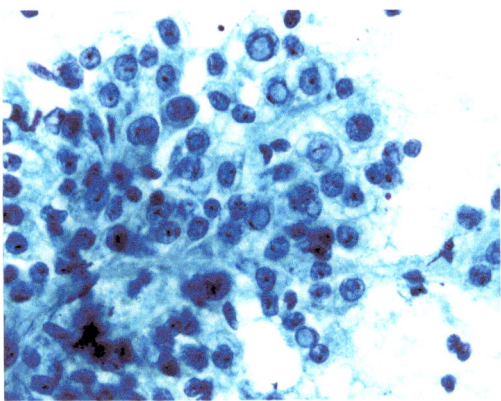

FIG. 3.28.   Hepatocellular Carcinoma, Intranuclear inclusions: These hepatocytes show enlarged nuclei with scattered irregular shapes and have prominent nucleoli. There are numerous intranuclear inclusions which are characteristic of HCC, but not specific as they can be seen in nonneoplastic processes. (Papanicolaou stain, high power)

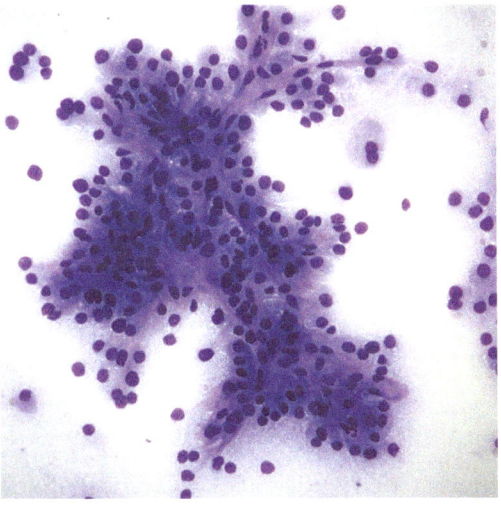

FIG. 3.29.   Hepatocellular Carcinoma, Well differentiated: A fragment of well-differentiated HCC with small transgressing blood vessels. There are scattered single cells in the background showing characteristic abundant granular cytoplasm and round nuclei. (Diff-Quik stain, medium power)

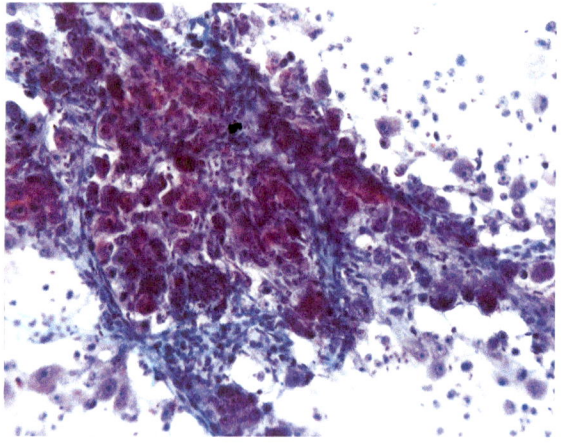

Fig. 3.30.   Hepatocellular Carcinoma, Moderately Differentiated: A fragment of neoplastic tissue showing hepatocytic differentiation is surrounded by endothelial cells with delicate spindled nuclei. The tumor cells show abundant granular cytoplasm and enlarged nuclei with very large nucleoli. These are features of a moderately differentiated hepatocellular carcinoma. (Papanicolaou stain, medium power)

Key features:

- Cellular aspirate
- Cellular fragments and numerous single cells
- Bare nuclei
- Cytomorphology similar to normal hepatocytes, losing differentiation with higher grade
- Absent bile ducts

Cytomorphology, HCC, Well Differentiated

Well-differentiated (WD) HCC is difficult to distinguish from nonneoplastic liver, and it is often challenging to make a diagnosis of malignancy on these samples (Figs. 3.27 and 3.29).

Key features:

- Hypercellular aspirate
- Predominantly fragments with loosely cohesive hepatocytes
- Scattered single cells
- Trabecular more than two cell thick
- Endothelial cells transgress fragments of hepatocytes
- Endothelial cells envelop groups of hepatocytes (endothelial wrapping or peripheral rimming)
- Granular cytoplasm
- Slight overall cellular enlargement
- Slightly increased n/c ratio
- Bare nuclei may be abundant
- Variable nucleoli
- Bile pigment—intracytoplasmic or intracanalicular

Cytomorphology, HCC, Moderately Differentiated

Moderately differentiated (MD) HCC shows features intermediate between well- and poorly differentiated HCC. It is readily recognized as malignant and shows enough hepatocytic differentiation that distinction from other primary or metastatic malignancies is not typically a challenge (Fig. 3.30).

Key features:

- Hypercellular aspirate
- Fragments with increased single cells (versus well differentiated)
- Increasing n/c ratio
- Numerous bare nuclei
- Prominent nucleoli
- Endothelial wrapping and transgressing vessels present, but less prominent than well differentiated

Cytomorphology, HCC, Poorly Differentiated

Poorly differentiated (PD) HCC is readily recognized as malignant, but is often difficult to pinpoint morphologically as hepatocytic in origin (Figs. 3.31 and 3.32).

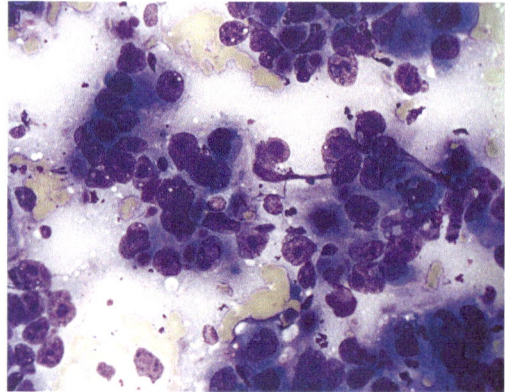

FIG. 3.31.   Hepatocellular Carcinoma, Poorly differentiated: This tumor consists of poorly differentiated tumor cells forming loose aggregates. The characteristic granular cytoplasm of HCC is not evident. The nuclei show anisonucleosis and macronucleoli. The differential diagnosis in this case would include metastatic malignant melanoma and poorly differentiated adenocarcinoma. (Diff-Quik stain, high power)

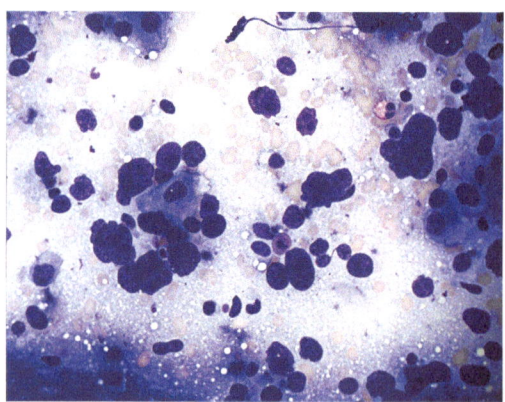

FIG. 3.32.   Hepatocellular Carcinoma, Poorly differentiated: These large, bare tumor nuclei show irregular nuclear contours and macronucleoli. There is little morphologic evidence to support a hepatocellular origin for these cells, thus immunostaining would be of great utility. (Diff-Quik stain, high power)

Key features:

- Hypercellular aspirate
- Marked variability in tumor size
- High n/c ratio
- Irregular nuclear shapes
- Thin nuclear membranes
- Prominent to enormous nucleoli
- Abundant bare nuclei
- Rare endothelial wrapping or transgressing vessels
- Tumor giant cells
- Cytoplasm may not show granularity

Special Types of Hepatocellular Carcinoma

Fibrolamellar HCC

Fibrolamellar (FL) HCC is a distinct subtype of HCC comprising 5 % of all HCC and occurring in a much younger patient population than conventional HCC (mean age 25 years versus 61 years for conventional HCC). It arises in a noncirrhotic liver, is not associated with classic risk factors for HCC, and AFP is normal. FL HCC typically presents as a large, solitary mass, usually in the left lobe of the liver, and a fibrous central scar may be seen on imaging. It is heterogeneously enhancing on CT, washes out on venous phase, and often shows central calcifications. FL HCC also shows characteristic histologic and cytomorphologic features. Histologically, fibrous tissue is prominent and forms a central scar in the tumor. Individual tumor cells are oncocytic and may show cytoplasmic pale bodies or hyaline globules. Cytomorphologically, tumor cells are singly dispersed and show abundant oxyphilic cytoplasm. Tumor cells are two to three times larger than normal hepatocytes, but nuclei are also enlarged resulting in maintained nuclear to cytoplasmic ratio. Intracytoplasmic "pale bodies" (dense eosinophilic material) are characteristic and often seen on aspirate smears (Fig. 3.33). Aspirates from FL HCC typically

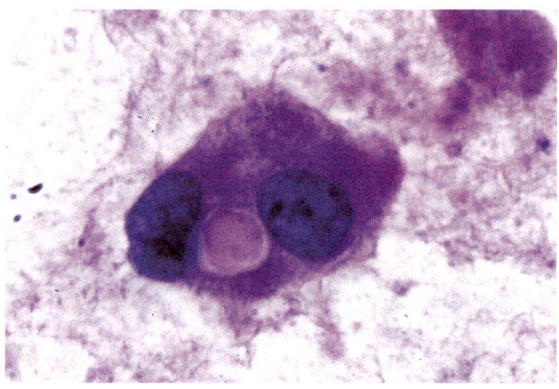

FIG. 3.33. Hepatocellular Carcinoma, Fibrolamellar type, pale body: This malignant hepatocyte shows a dense eosinophilic structure in the cytoplasm (between the two nuclei) representing a pale body. This is characteristic of fibrolamellar type HCC. (Diff-Quik stain, high power)

lack peripheral endothelial wrapping, but may have transgressing vessels. Dense fibrous bands suggest the diagnosis (Figs. 3.34 and 3.35).

Key features:

- Monotonous, predominantly single cells
- Abundant dense oxyphilic cytoplasm
- Intranuclear inclusions
- Intracytoplasmic "pale bodies" (dense eosinophilic material)
- Lack endothelial wrapping, but may have transgressing vessels
- Dense fibrous bands

Differential diagnosis:

Depending on the grade of HCC, the differential diagnosis varies. WD HCC should be distinguished from regenerative nodules or dysplastic nodules in cirrhosis, which typically show lower cellularity, normal (low) nuclear to cytoplasmic ratio, focal rather than monotonous atypia, none to small nucleoli and single cells, or monolayers arranged as thin cords

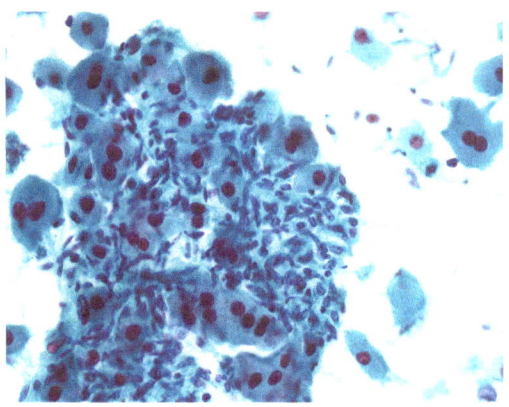

FIG. 3.34.   Hepatocellular Carcinoma, Fibrolamellar type: Dense fibrous tissue surrounds small clusters of malignant hepatocytes. There are scattered single cells present in the background. These hepatocytes are atypical, showing nuclear enlargement and irregular nuclear contours. There is intimately admixed fibrous tissue with small   bland spindled nuclei characteristic of fibrolamellar HCC (Papanicolaou stain, high power)

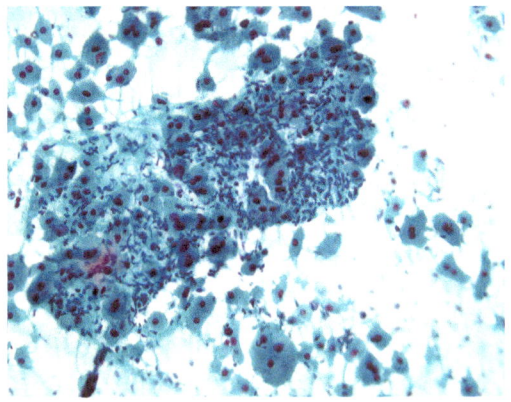

FIG. 3.35.   Hepatocellular Carcinoma, Fibrolamellar type: Atypical hepatocytes, many of which are binucleated are embedded in dense fibrous tissue. There are many scattered malignant hepatocytes present in the background. (Papanicolaou stain, intermediate power)

(one to two cells thick). In addition, liver cell adenoma or focal nodular hyperplasia (FNH) is in the differential with WD HCC, but should not show numerous single cells or abnormal vascular patterns. The radiographic appearance and background liver status (i.e., cirrhosis) are also important clues to the diagnosis. Angiomyolipoma should be considered in the differential diagnosis of WD HCC as it can show epithelioid and or spindle cells with granular cytoplasm and numerous blood vessels. Typically the architecture is that of sheets of epithelioid cells with scattered bizarre cells. Immunostains for HMB45 and SMA are positive in angiomyolipoma and confirm the diagnosis. A number of metastatic malignancies are in the differential diagnosis for HCC and are discussed in more detail at the end of this chapter. Briefly, adrenal cortical carcinoma is considered in the differential for WD HCC, particularly because it can show endothelial wrapping on tissue sections. Renal cell carcinoma is considered in the differential for WD and MD HCC. A broad group of malignancies, including malignant melanoma, neuroendocrine tumors, epithelioid gastrointestinal stromal tumor (GIST), and adenocarcinoma from pancreas, colon, and lung are considered in the differential for MD and PD HCC. Immunostains can be helpful and are necessary in some cases. Detailed immunohistochemical differentiation is discussed later in this chapter.

Immunohistochemical studies and special stains on CB or NCB:

A reticulin special stain is of great utility in assessing hepatocytic proliferations on CB or NCB. HCC shows a loss of or absence of reticulin framework and highlights thickened trabeculae, greater than three cells thick. A number of immunohistochemical studies can be performed to confirm hepatocytic origin and to help distinguish nonmalignant hepatocytic populations from HCC, though no marker is entirely diagnostic (Table 3.3). Hepatocyte Paraffin 1 (HepPar1) is the most sensitive and specific marker for HCC (both >80 %). It shows diffuse granular cytoplasmic staining in HCC, but is also positive in normal hepatocytes and hepatic adenomas, so it is not

TABLE 3.3.   Immunohistochemical and special stains useful in the diagnosis of HCC.

* Reticulin
  – Loss of or absence of reticulin framework
  – Thickened trabeculae, greater than 3 cells thick
* HepPar1
  – Most sensitive and specific marker for HCC (both >80 %)
  – Diffuse granular cytoplasmic staining
  – More often negative in poorly differentiated or sclerosing HCC
  – Patchy staining is seen in 20 % of HCC
* Carcinoembryonic antigen, polyclonal (pCEA)
  – Canalicular pattern of expression in 60–90 % of HCC
    – Sensitivity >80 % in well and moderately differentiated HCC
    – Lower sensitivity (25–50 %) in poorly differentiated HCC
* Cytokeratins 7 and 20
  – Most HCCs are CK7–/CK20–
  – 20 % are CK7+/CK20–
  – 5 % are CK7+/CK20+
* CD34
  – Not expressed in sinusoids of normal liver
  – Strongly expressed in sinusoids in HCC
    – Highly specific
    – Low sensitivity (20–40 %)
  – Most useful in distinguishing well-differentiated HCC from normal liver or cirrhosis, particularly in small biopsy samples

helpful in distinguishing HCC from normal and reactive processes. HepPar1 is negative or very focally positive in most adenocarcinomas, melanoma, and epithelioid angiomyolipoma, all of which often enter into the differential diagnosis of HCC, though strong staining can be seen in some cases of gastric, esophageal, lung, and pancreatic (rare) adenocarcinomas. It is more often negative in poorly differentiated or sclerosing HCC, and patchy staining is seen in 20 % of HCC, so interpretation in small CB or NCB samples must be performed in conjunction with a panel of other immunostains.

Polyclonal carcinoembryonic antigen (pCEA) shows a distinct canalicular pattern of expression in 60–90 % of HCC (Fig. 3.36). The sensitivity is greater than 80 % in well- and moderately differentiated HCC, but is lower (25–50 %) in poorly differentiated HCC. Diffuse cytoplasmic positivity is seen in most adenocarcinomas (>90 %), so noting the pattern

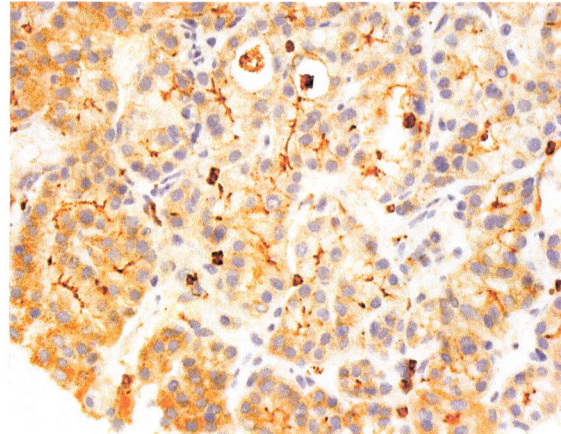

Fig. 3.36.   Hepatocellular carcinoma: Polyclonal CEA produces a characteristic canalicular staining pattern in hepatocellular carcinoma that is not seen in adenocarcinomas. (Core biopsy, pCEA immunostain, medium power)

of expression is essential to its utility. pCEA does not distinguish HCC from benign hepatocellular nodules. Both CD10 and villin produce a similar canalicular pattern of staining to pCEA in HCC, but have much lower sensitivity and are not of great utility.

The vascular marker CD34 is not expressed in sinusoids of normal liver, but is strongly expressed in sinusoids in HCC (Fig. 3.37). It is highly specific for HCC, but shows a low sensitivity (20–40 %). It has greatest utility in distinguishing well-differentiated HCC from normal liver or cirrhosis, particularly in small biopsy samples.

Glypican 3 is a relatively new immunohistochemical marker normally expressed in fetal liver and placenta, but not in normal adult liver or hepatic adenoma. It is expressed in 64–90 % of HCC, and thus is highly sensitive (>80 %) for HCC. In particular, it has a higher sensitivity for poorly differentiated HCC than HepPar1. It is also positive in some high grade dysplastic nodules, so positivity does not assure

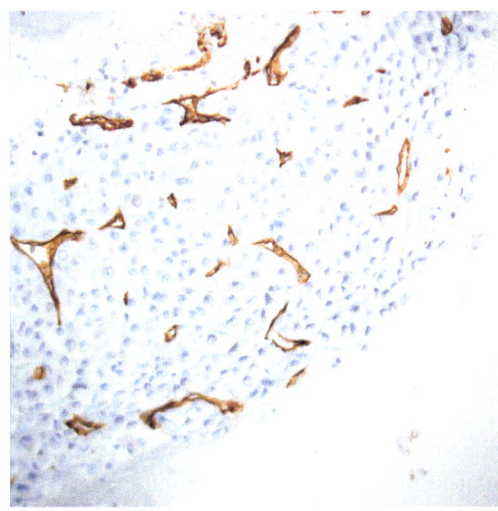

FIG. 3.37.   Hepatocellular carcinoma: CD34 does not react with normal sinusoids in the liver; the presence of this positive sinusoidal pattern is suspicious for hepatocellular carcinoma. This can be particularly useful on small CB or NCB samples. (Core biopsy, CD34 immunostain, medium power)

malignancy, and it is also expressed in melanoma and nonseminomatous germ cell tumors (yolk sac tumor and choriocarcinoma). As this marker is relatively new, further studies are needed to confirm its efficacy in the setting of HCC.

Alpha-fetoprotein (AFP) is expressed by HCC and yolk sac tumors, but immunostaining is patchy or negative. It has a low sensitivity (30–50 %) and a high specificity (exclude germ cell tumors), but is overall not useful for the primary diagnosis of HCC. Moc-31 is positive in most (80–90 %) adenocarcinomas, including cholangiocarcinoma (diffuse membranous positivity) but most HCCs are negative or weakly positive. Cytokeratins (CK) can be useful in the diagnosis of HCC. CK8 and CK18 and Cam 5.2 are usually positive in normal and neoplastic hepatocytes, as well as HCC. AE1/3 cytokeratin cocktail is typically patchy or negative. The most common immunostaining pattern for CK7 and

CK20 is CK7–/CK20–, but 20 % are CK7+/CK20– and 5 % are CK7+/CK20+. CK19 is positive in 85–100 % of cholangio-carcinoma, but is negative or patchy in HCC.

Intrahepatic Cholangiocarcinoma

The second most common primary hepatic malignancy after HCC is intrahepatic cholangiocarcinoma (IC), comprising 10–20 % of primary hepatic malignancies. ICs arise in noncir-rhotic liver and have a poor prognosis. Treatment is surgical resection, but the vast majority of the tumors are unresect-able at diagnosis. Risk factors include parasitic infection (*Clonorchis sinensis*, *Opisthorchis viverrini*), primary scleros-ing cholangitis (PSC), choledochal cysts, Caroli syndrome, cholelithiasis, and Thorotrast exposure. PSC is the most important causative factor in the Western world. Six to thirty-six percent of patients with PSC develop cholangiocar-cinoma, thus those patients are routinely monitored by serial ERCP-directed bile duct brushings. Forty to sixty per-cent of cholangiocarcinomas are hilar, 10–15 % are intrahe-patic (peripheral), and the remainder are extrahepatic. Histologically, ICs show malignant glands with intracytoplas-mic mucin and a background of prominent desmoplasia (Fig. 3.38). Bile is absent. Aspirate smears are hypercellular and often show well-differentiated glandular structures. Smears show predominantly tissue fragments with disorga-nized monolayer sheets or an acinar pattern. Nuclear to cytoplasmic ratios are high (much higher than WD and MD HCC), and there are variable nucleoli (Figs. 3.39 and 3.40). A mucin stain may highlight intracytoplasmic mucin vacu-oles (Fig. 3.41).

Key features:

- Hypercellular aspirate
- Predominantly tissue fragments with disorganized mono-layer sheets or acinar pattern
- High n/c ratio
- Variable nucleoli

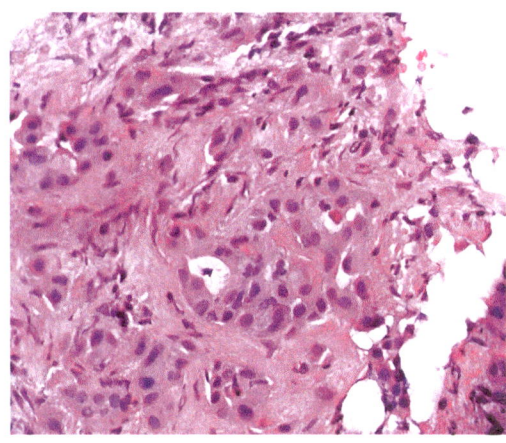

FIG. 3.38.   Cholangiocarcinoma: This small core biopsy specimen shows small glandular structures surrounded by desmoplastic stroma. While there are no specific immunomarkers for cholangiocarcinoma, immunostains may be performed to rule out metastatic adenocarcinoma from other sites, depending on the clinical and radiographic impression. (Core biopsy, H&E stain, high power)

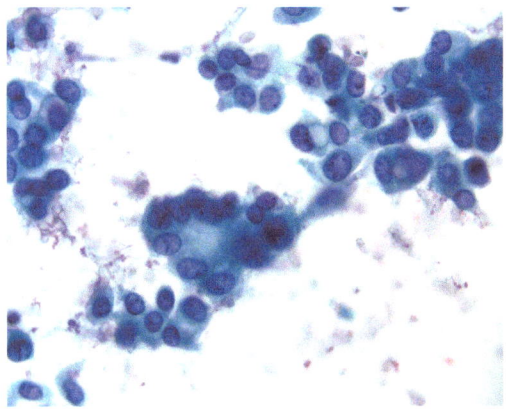

FIG. 3.39.   Cholangiocarcinoma: An acinar structure is shown in the *center* of the field illustrating glandular differentiation. In addition, several cells (1 and 2 o'clock) show intracytoplasmic mucin vacuoles also supporting glandular differentiation. Cholangiocarcinoma cannot be morphologically distinguished from metastatic adenocarcinoma. (Papanicolaou stain, high power)

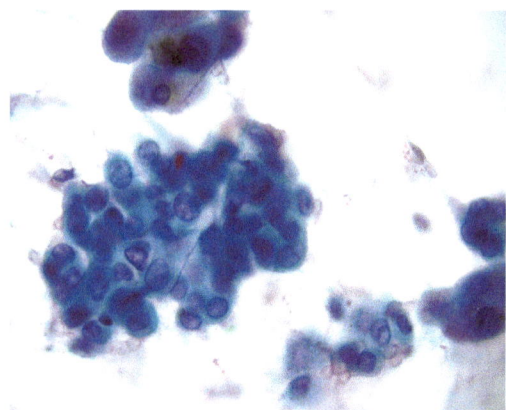

Fig. 3.40. Cholangiocarcinoma: A very disorganized fragment of glandular epithelium is present in the *center* of the field showing nuclear overlap and crowding. The nuclear to cytoplasmic ratio is high and the nuclear contours are irregular. Vague glandular formations can be appreciated, indicating adenocarcinoma. A group of benign hepatocytes is present in the *upper portion* of the image for comparison. (Papanicolaou stain, high power)

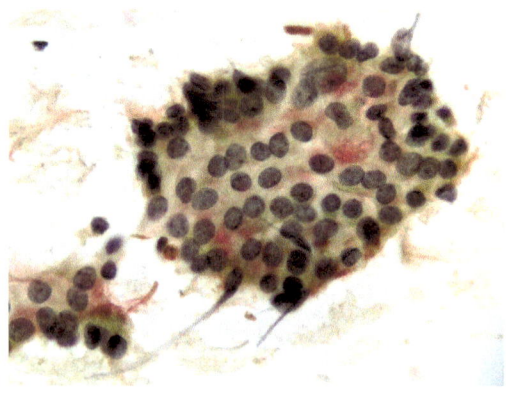

Fig. 3.41. Cholangiocarcinoma: This mucicarmine stain highlights cytoplasmic mucin (*bright pink*), supporting the diagnosis of adenocarcinoma. This stain may be helpful in differentiating poorly differentiated adenocarcinoma from hepatocellular carcinoma. (Mucicarmine stain, medium power)

Differential diagnosis:
The most common differential diagnosis for IC is metastatic adenocarcinoma, but IC cannot be distinguished cytomorphologically or immunohistochemically from metastatic adenocarcinoma originating in the pancreas or extrahepatic biliary system. Correlation with clinical and radiographic findings is essential. Less commonly, the differential includes HCC with an acinar pattern and shows features of hepatocytic differentiation including abundant granular cytoplasm and prominent nucleoli.

Also see Chap. 4 for a discussion of bile duct brushings for cholangiocarcinoma

Combined HCC/Cholangiocarcinoma

Combined HCC and IC is a rare diagnostic entity. In order to make the diagnosis, there must be demonstration of a distinct population of HCC and cholangiocarcinoma as well as a transitional component between the two populations.

Rare Primary Malignant Neoplasms

Hematopoietic Malignancies

Primary hematopoietic malignancies of the liver are morphologically identical to those originating in other sites (primary or metastatic). Large B-cell lymphoma and Hodgkin lymphoma are the most commonly encountered lymphomas primary to the liver. Aspirates from non-Hodgkin lymphoma, such as low grade B-cell lymphomas, are cellular and show a monomorphic population of dispersed, single cells with lymphoglandular bodies present in background. Higher grade B-cell lymphomas show a dispersed population of variably atypical single cells with basophilic cytoplasm and often have nucleoli and prominent mitotic activity. Hodgkin lymphoma is characterized by Reed-Sternberg cells most often in a mixed inflammatory background that includes eosinophils.

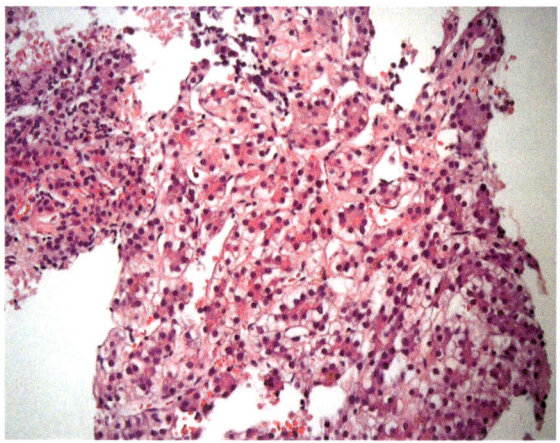

Fɪɢ. 3.42.   Hepatoblastoma: This cell block preparation shows a population of neoplastic cells with an appearance of immature liver. Groups of fetal-type hepatocytes form small aggregates surrounded by sinusoids. The nuclear to cytoplasmic ratio is higher than in mature hepatocytes and the cytoplasm is slightly less granular. Nuclear atypia is not marked. (H&E stain, low power)

Hepatoblastoma

Hepatoblastoma (HB) is the most common primary malignant liver tumor in children and comprises approximately half of all malignant pediatric hepatic tumors. Over 60 % occur in children under age 2, and 90 % occur before age 5. The average age at the time of diagnosis is 18 months. HBs are associated with Beckwith-Wiedemann syndrome, Down syndrome, and familial polyposis coli. Clinically, patients present with a large palpable abdominal mass, hepatomegaly, abdominal pain, and fever. Serum AFP is elevated in 90 % of cases, and 50–90 % of the tumors have an associated β-catenin mutation. Radiographically, HB is a solitary mass, more often in right lobe of the liver. Treatment includes resection and chemotherapy. Histologically, HB is separated into three subtypes: epithelial, mixed, and small cell (anaplastic). The epithelial type is the most common, comprising 60 % of all HB, and shows a combination of fetal and embryonal cells (Fig. 3.42). The fetal cells resemble normal hepatocytes, but are smaller and are arranged in plates or cords. The embryonal cells are primitive with hyperchromatic nuclei and scant cytoplasm and may form rosettes and trabeculae. The mixed subtype comprises 30 % of HB and consists of epithelial and mesenchymal components. The epithelial component is described above, and the mesenchymal component consists of spindle cells with heterologous elements including skeletal muscle, osteoid, chondroid elements, calcification, and extramedullary hematopoiesis. The least common subtype of HB, small-cell (anaplastic), accounts for 10 % of HB and shows monomorphous cells with scant cytoplasm and a high mitotic rate. They resemble other small round blue cell tumors.

Aspirates of HB show abundant cellularity. The epithelial component is typically the most prominent, though the morphologic appearance depends on the tumor subtype. Most commonly, epithelial cells are arranged in three-dimensional clusters (acini), trabeculae, sheets, and rosettes. The fetal type of HB shows cellular aspirates with well-formed acini having low nuclear to cytoplasmic ratio, round to oval nuclei with finely granular chromatin, inconspicuous nucleoli, and abundant cytoplasm. Cytoplasmic and nuclear vacuoles may be prominent. Embryonal types show more sheets, clusters, and rosettes and have higher nuclear to cytoplasmic ratios with hyperchromatic nuclei and conspicuous nucleoli. Mesenchymal elements (osteoid, cartilage, skeletal muscle) are less abundant on aspirate smears than the epithelial component (Figs. 3.43, 3.44, 3.45, 3.46, and 3.47). Anaplastic tumors produce smears containing immature, small blue cells with mitoses and karyorrhexis in a background of necrosis. The background in any subtype may also show acellular eosinophilic material, focal necrosis, extramedullary hematopoiesis, or nucleated red blood cells.

Key features:

- Abundant cellularity
- Epithelial cells arranged in:
  - Acini (most common)
  - Trabeculae
  - Sheets
  - Rosettes

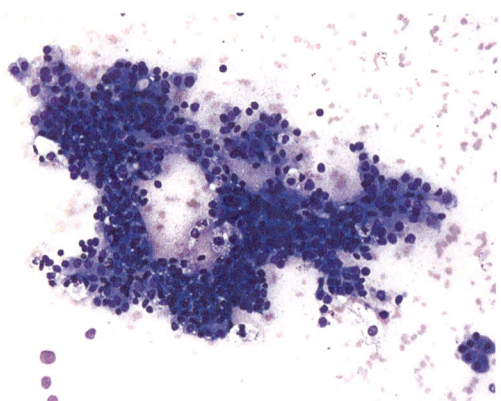

FIG. 3.43.   Hepatoblastoma: A cohesive sheet of tumor cells is shown with increased nuclear to cytoplasmic ratios. Most nuclei are round to oval with smooth nuclear contours and only focal pleomorphism. Small spindle-shaped nuclei representing endothelial cells are embedded with the neoplastic epithelial cells. (Diff-Quik stain, medium power)

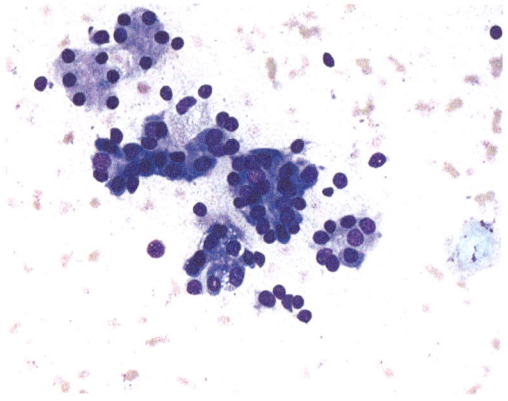

FIG. 3.44.   Hepatoblastoma: The cells present in the *center* of the image are immature hepatocytes which show large nuclei and high nuclear to cytoplasmic ratios. There is a group of mature hepatocytes present at 11 o'clock for comparison. They show similar overall cell size, but smaller, round nuclei and thus a lower nuclear to cytoplasmic ratio. (Diff-Quik stain, high power)

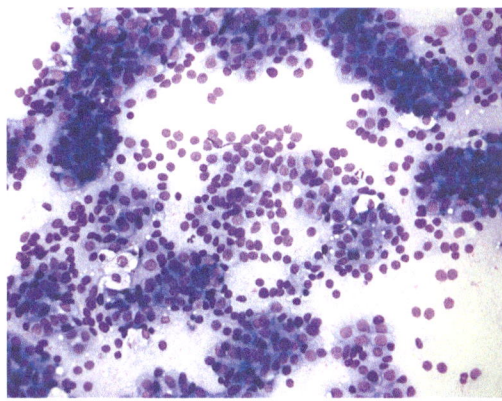

FIG. 3.45.   Hepatoblastoma: The neoplastic cells shown here show vague acinar formations but are loosely cohesive and there are some single cells in the background, as well as some bare nuclei. Hepatocellular carcinoma is in the differential diagnosis, though the cytoplasm is less granular and the nuclear to cytoplasmic ratio is higher than in HCC. (Diff-Quik stain, medium power)

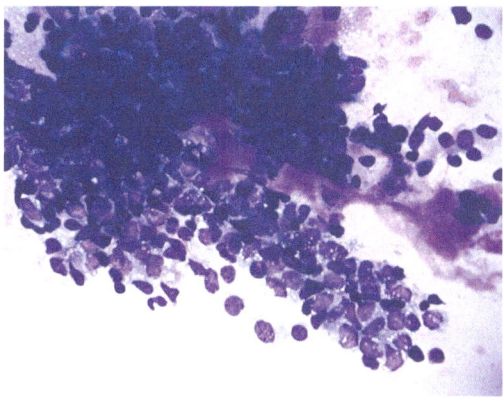

FIG. 3.46.   Hepatoblastoma: These tumor cells show a very high nuclear to cytoplasmic ratio and have angulated nuclei. There is matrix material (eosinophilic, fibrillary) present, which may be seen in hepatoblastoma. The differential would include other small round cell neoplasms or mesenchymal tumors. (Diff-Quik stain, medium power)

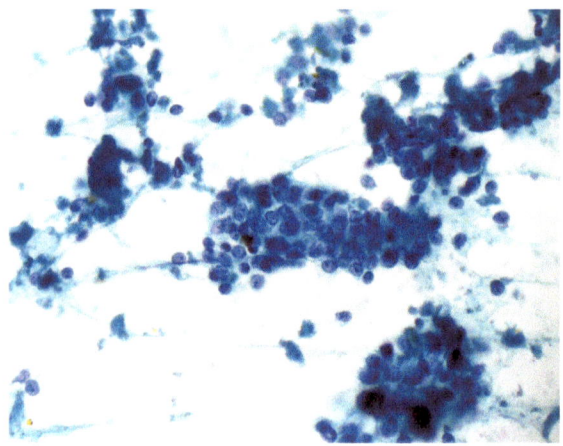

Fɪɢ. 3.47.   Hepatoblastoma: A fragment of neoplastic epithelium is present in the center of the field and shows very high nuclear to cytoplasmic ratios. The chromatin is evenly dispersed and there are no prominent nucleoli. Adenocarcinoma would be considered in the differential diagnosis in this case, though that diagnosis would be uncommon in the young age group. (Papanicolaou stain, medium power)

- Round to oval epithelial cells
- Moderate pleomorphism
- Low n/c ratio
- Finely granular chromatin
- Small nucleoli
- Mesenchymal component less common on smears

  - Eosinophilic acellular stroma
  - Clusters of bland spindle cells

- Background

  - Acellular eosinophilic material
  - Focal necrosis
  - Extramedullary hematopoiesis
  - Nucleated red blood cells

Differential diagnosis:
Hepatocellular carcinoma is more common than HB, even in the pediatric age group, and it is at the top of the differential diagnosis list. In the absence of a mesenchymal component, which favors HB, the epithelial component should show more immature features. In addition, HBs tend to stain for high molecular weight CK, but most HCCs are negative. Other pediatric small round blue cell tumors also enter into the differential diagnosis, including Wilms tumor and neuroblastoma, but clinical and radiographic correlation can often assist in the diagnosis.

Undifferentiated (Embryonal) Sarcoma

Undifferentiated sarcoma is the third most common primary hepatic tumor in children, but it is very rare. It is most common in children ages 6–10 years old. Histologically, tumors show anaplastic cells with marked pleomorphism. Some tumor cells are spindled and others are very large with abundant eosinophilic cytoplasm containing PAS positive hyaline globules.

Morphologically, aspirate smears are usually hypercellular and show atypical spindle cells and often bizarre pleomorphic tumor cells. Both intracytoplasmic and extracellular eosinophilic globules are characteristic and a PAS positive. There is a variable amount of myxoid stroma present in the background (Figs. 3.48, 3.49, 3.50, and 3.51).

Key features:

- Usually hypercellular aspirates
- Atypical spindle cells, bizarre pleomorphic tumor cells
- Variable amount of myxoid stroma
- Intracytoplasmic and extracellular eosinophilic globules (d-PAS+)

Angiosarcoma

Angiosarcoma (AS) represents less than 1 % of primary hepatic malignancies. The tumor affects males more often than females, typically in the age range of 60–70 years.

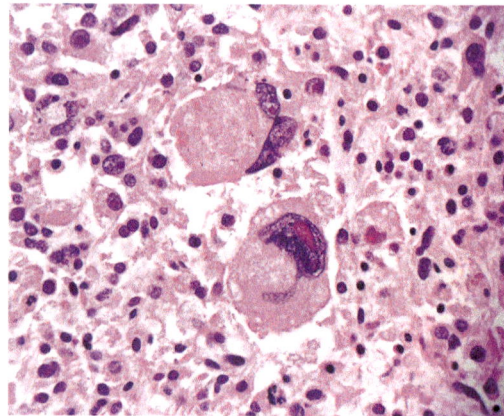

FIG. 3.48.   Embryonal Sarcoma: Two enormous malignant cells are present in the *center* of the field which show irregularly, shaped angulated nuclei with prominent nucleoli. The surrounding malignant cells also show angulated nuclei with very prominent nucleoli. (Cell block, H&E stain, medium power)

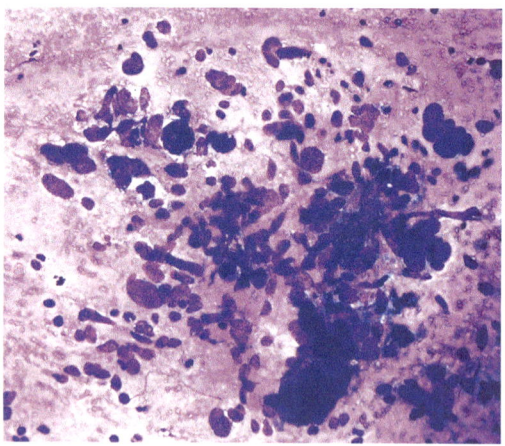

FIG. 3.49.   Embryonal Sarcoma: Marked anisonucleosis with very irregular nuclear shapes is evident in this aspirate smear. Some of the smaller cells show a spindle shape, indicating mesenchymal differentiation. There is eosinophilic matrix present in the background. (Diff-Quik stain, medium power)

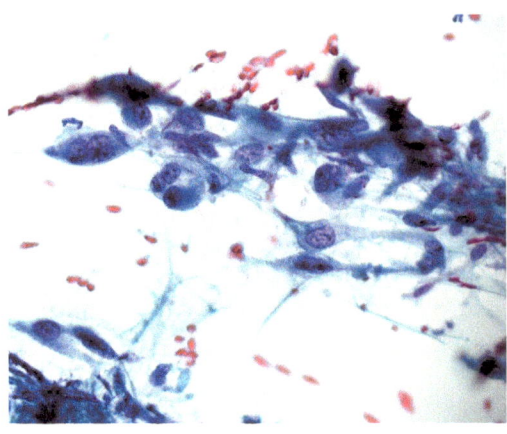

FIG. 3.50.   Embryonal Sarcoma: These malignant cells show a spindled morphology with marked nuclear atypia including irregular chromatin distribution and anisonucleosis. (Papanicolaou stain, high power)

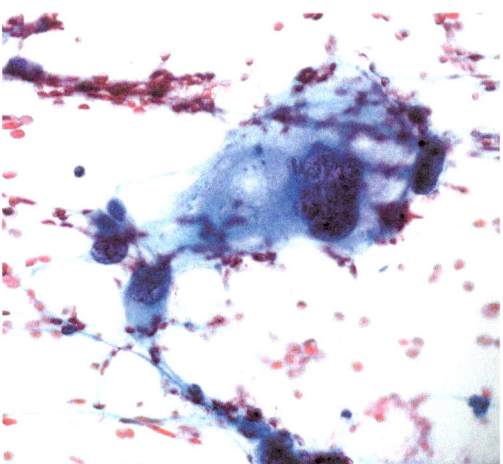

FIG. 3.51.   Embryonal Sarcoma: A bizarre multinucleated tumor cells is present with a few smaller tumor cells surrounding it. This degree of pleomorphism is consistent with a high-grade sarcoma. (Papanicolaou stain, high power)

It is associated with cirrhosis, polyvinyl chloride, arsenic, and Thorotrast exposure. Clinical presentation includes hepato-megaly, ascites, and abdominal pain. CT scan shows either single or multiple masses with irregular outlines. The progno-sis for AS is poor with mean survival of 6 months. Histologic sections show anastomosing vascular channels lined by endo-thelial cells with variable pleomorphism, which may either be hobnail epithelioid cells or spindle cells. If AS is suspected clinically or radiographically, FNA may be avoided as hemor-rhage is a potential complication. If aspirated, smears are typically blood and may be hypercellular. Either spindled or epithelioid endothelial cells, similar to those seen histologically, are present. There is often pleomorphism and multinucle-ation. Vascular markers such as CD34 and CD31 should be positive on CB or NCB preparations.

Key features:

- Bloody smears
- Fragments and single cells
- Atypical endothelial cells
  - Spindled
  - Epithelioid

- Pleomorphism

Differential diagnosis:

Depending on the degree of differentiation in the AS, the dif-ferential diagnosis includes other vascular tumors such as epithelioid hemangioendothelioma (ES) (discussed below) which is a lower grade vascular tumor, and metastatic sarcomas, which typically show higher nuclear grade and pleomorphism. Vascular immunostains may help differenti-ate AS from a metastatic nonvascular sarcoma.

Epithelioid Hemangioendothelioma

Epithelioid hemangioendothelioma (ES) is a rare, low-grade vascular tumor that may be seen in a number of organs, including liver. It affects patients over a wide age range (20–80 years) and is associated with exposure to oral contraceptives as well as polyvinyl chloride. Aspirates of ES show scant cellularity with scattered spindle cells exhibiting prominent nucleoli and occasional intracytoplasmic lumina, characteristic of ES. Rarely, pleomorphic cells and multinucleated tumor cells may be seen.

Key features:

- Scant cellularity
- Prominent nucleoli
- Occasional intracytoplasmic lumina

Metastatic Neoplasms to Liver

Approximately one quarter of all metastases to solid organs are found in the liver, making it one of the most common sites for metastatic disease. By far, the most common metastatic lesions are carcinomas, though melanomas, sarcomas, and lymphomas are all seen as metastatic liver lesions. In the noncirrhotic liver, metastases are approximately 30 times more common than hepatocellular carcinoma.

Metastatic malignancies may originate from any site and typically present as multiple nodules (80 % of cases), generally involving both hepatic lobes. Correlation with clinical history and radiographic findings is essential, though metastatic tumors may sometimes be detected in a patient with no known primary. Whenever possible, material should be obtained for CB or NCB preparation to allow for immunostaining to determine the primary site.

Metastatic Carcinomas

The most common metastatic tumor type is adenocarcinoma, which can be from any primary site but is most commonly from (in order of decreasing frequency) lung, colon, pancreas, breast, stomach, ovary, prostate, or endometrium (Table 3.4). Additional metastatic carcinoma types include squamous cell carcinoma (SqCC), which is uncommon and may be from head and neck, genital, anorectal, lung, or esophagus. The morphology of the

TABLE 3.4.   Common primary sites for metastatic adenocarcinoma to liver.

- Lung (25 %)
- Colon (16 %)
- Pancreas (11 %)
- Breast (10 %)
- Stomach (6 %)

TABLE 3.5   Differentiation of carcinoma metastases based on CK7 and CK20 immunohistochemistry.

	CK7+	CK7–
CK20+	Pancreas/biliary tract Urothelial carcinoma Esophagus/stomach Ovary (Mucinous) Lung (Mucinous bronchioloalveolar)	Colorectal
CK20–	Breast Lung Pancreas/biliary tract Endometrium Esophagus/stomach Ovary (nonmucinous)	Hepatocellular carcinoma Prostatic carcinoma Renal Cell carcinoma Adrenal Cortical carcinoma

SqCC does not indicate the primary site. Keratinization is helpful when seen on aspirate smears, but it is not always present. Urothelial carcinoma shows a predominant single cell pattern with round to oval nuclei having occasional nuclear grooves and eccentric nuclei with cytoplasmic "tails." Renal cell carcinoma may metastasize to the liver, though the lung is a more common site, and shows typical clear cell features such as vacuolated cytoplasm, ill-defined cell borders, and prominent nucleoli. In the differentiation of metastatic carcinomas, CK7 and CK20 can be helpful (Table 3.5).

Key features:

- Columnar cells forming acinar structures with central lumina
- Varying degrees of nuclear atypia
- Prominent nucleoli common

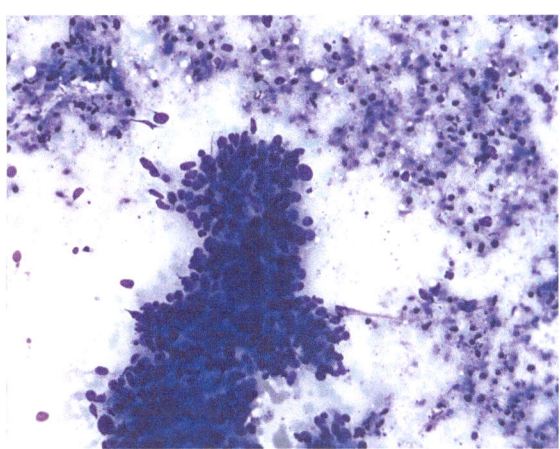

Fɪɢ. 3.52.   Metastatic colonic adenocarcinoma: A cohesive cluster of malignant cells is shown with some nuclear elongation and columnar arrangement present at the edge of the fragment. The background shows granular necrotic debris. These findings are characteristic of metastatic colon cancer. (Diff-Quik stain, medium power)

- Typically focal mucin production (cytoplasmic, luminal, or extracellular)
- Background necrosis, depending on primary site (colon, pancreas)

In some cases, the morphology may favor a specific primary site, though the clinical history and immunostaining profile are typically most helpful in establishing a primary site. Metastatic colonic adenocarcinoma can often be recognized by its necrotic "grungy" background admixed with malignant tall columnar cells with cigar-shaped nuclei (Figs. 3.52, 3.53, 3.54, and 3.55). Metastases from other sites, including pancreas, can show a background of necrosis, so this finding is not specific for colonic adenocarcinoma. Pancreaticobiliary neoplasms often show focal to abundant desmoplastic stroma, which may suggest the primary (Figs. 3.56 and 3.57). Breast carcinoma, particularly lobular

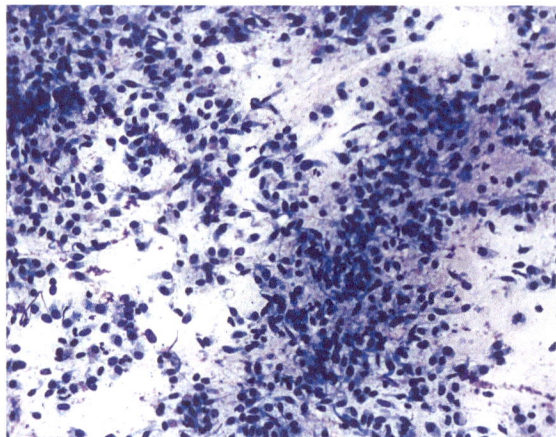

FIG. 3.53.   Metastatic colonic adenocarcinoma: Numerous columnar shaped malignant cells are present in a granular background.
Though fragments of cohesive malignant cells are more common,
colonic adenocarcinoma may also present in this way. (Diff-Quik
stain, low power)

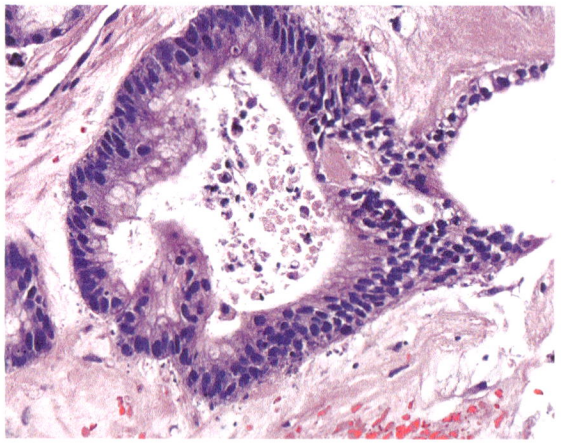

FIG. 3.54.   Metastatic colonic adenocarcinoma: A small core biopsy
captured a malignant glandular formation with elongated nuclei and
central necrosis. This biopsy is from the same case as Fig. 3.53 in
which mostly single cells were present. (H&E stain, medium power)

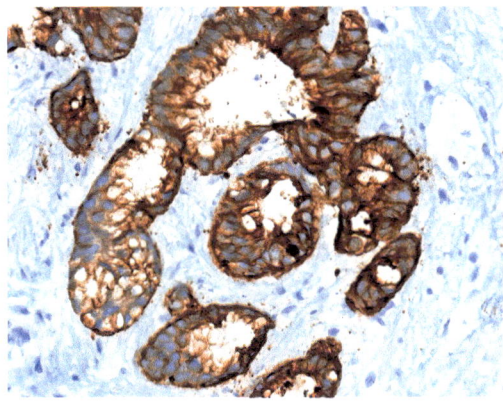

FIG. 3.55.   Metastatic colonic adenocarcinoma: The glandular formations shown here are strongly positive for Cytokeratin 20, supporting a colorectal primary. This patient had a history of colon cancer and multiple liver lesions. (CK20 immunostain, medium power)

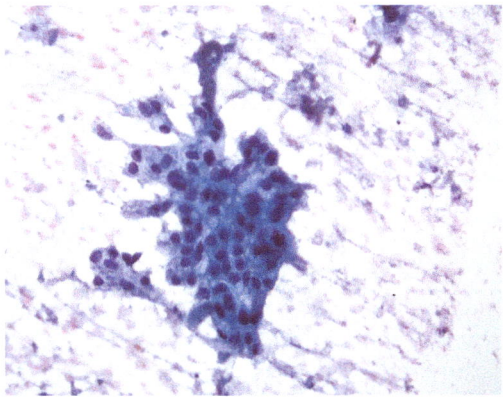

FIG. 3.56.   Metastatic pancreatic adenocarcinoma: An epithelial tissue fragment which shows a disorganized honeycomb architecture as well as anisonucleosis, consistent with a well-differentiated adenocarcinoma. There is also a necrotic background, which is sometimes seen in metastatic pancreatic carcinoma. (Papanicolaou stain, medium power)

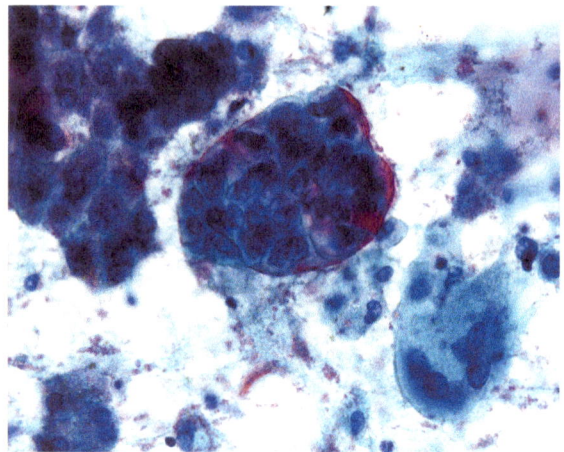

FIG. 3.57. Metastatic pancreatic adenocarcinoma: A group of malignant glandular cells with very high nuclear to cytoplasmic ratios and irregular nuclear contours is present in the *center* of the field. A group of benign hepatocytes is present in the *upper left*. The patient had a known history of pancreatic adenocarcinoma. (Papanicolaou stain, high power)

type, but also ductal type, may show numerous single cells, some of which have intracytoplasmic lumina (Figs. 3.58 and 3.59). Gastric carcinoma may show signet ring features, single cells with a single cytoplasmic mucin vacuole that displaces and compresses the nucleus to the periphery of the cell. These features are not specific to stomach, though, as they can occur anywhere in the gastrointestinal tract and can be difficult to differentiate from lobular breast carcinoma as well. Prostatic adenocarcinoma may show small acinar formations and prominent nucleoli. Metastatic papillary thyroid carcinoma often shows intranuclear inclusions, oval nuclei, and longitudinal nuclear grooves (Fig. 3.60), though these features may have some overlap with bronchioloalveolar type lung carcinoma. TTF1 and PAX-8 immunostaining may be very helpful in demonstrating thyroid origin (Fig. 3.61). Adenosquamous carcinoma (Fig. 3.62) shows features of both adenocarcinoma and at least a 30 % squamous component,

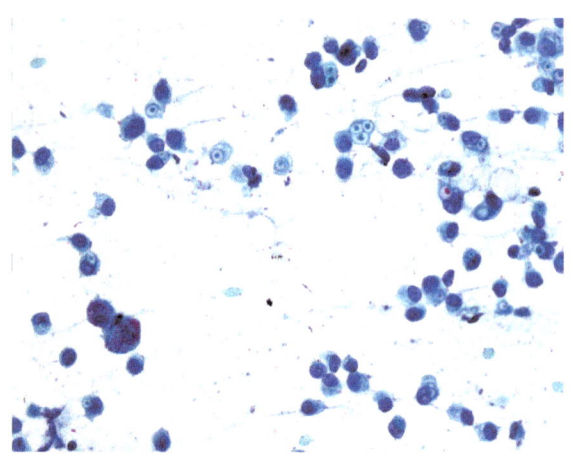

Fɪɢ. 3.58.   Metastatic mammary carcinoma, lobular type: There are numerous singly dispersed tumor cells present in this image and two hepatocytes are present at 8 o'clock for comparison. The nuclei of the tumor cells are approximately the same size as the hepatocyte nuclei. The tumor cells show eccentric nuclei and many show a distinct intracytoplasmic vacuole or lumen, characteristic of lobular breast carcinoma. (Papanicolaou stain, medium power)

though the percentage of squamous differentiation can be difficult to discern from aspirate smears. Possible primary sites include pancreas and biliary system, as well as other gastrointestinal sites and lung. Renal cell carcinoma (RCC) accounts for 3 % of all metastases to liver. The cytomorphology of conventional, clear cell carcinoma is quite characteristic and shows large, polygonal cells with abundant clear cytoplasm and ill-defined cell borders arranged singly and in clusters. Small blood vessels are often prominent and arranged in a transgressing pattern, though endothelial wrapping is not seen, which helps distinguish RCC from HCC. Nuclei are round with prominent nucleoli (Figs. 3.63 and 3.64). Immunohistochemically, RCCs are negative for HepPar1 and pCEA, but are positive for PAX-8, CD10, vimentin, EMA, and RCC (most clear cell and papillary types). PAX-2 is positive in 70–80 % of metastatic clear cell RCC. Though a rare

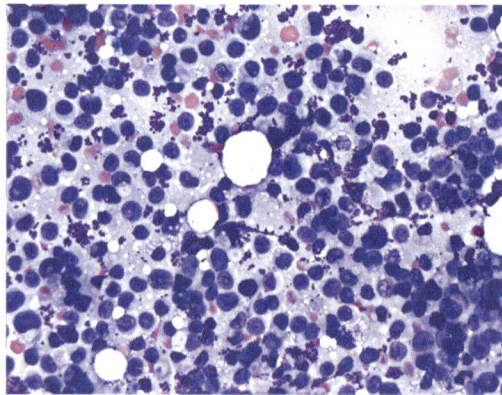

FIG. 3.59.   Metastatic mammary carcinoma, lobular type: This Diff Quik preparation corresponds to the Papanicolaou stained material in Fig. 3.58. The intracytoplasmic vacuoles are more difficult to appreciate, though they are present. The tumor cells are rather monotonous and singly dispersed. A neuroendocrine tumor could be considered in the differential diagnosis given the uniformity of the tumor cells, though the cytoplasmic vacuole would favor and adenocarcinoma. (Diff-Quik stain, high power)

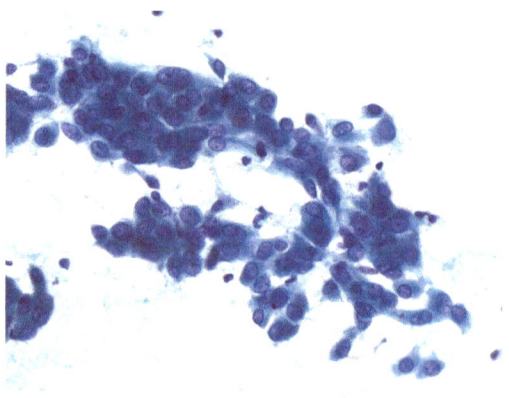

FIG. 3.60.   Metastatic papillary thyroid carcinoma: This group of neoplastic cells is forming a cohesive flat sheet. The nuclei are predominantly oval shaped and show an inclusion (6 o'clock). Adenocarcinoma would be considered in the differential. (Papanicolaou stain, medium power)

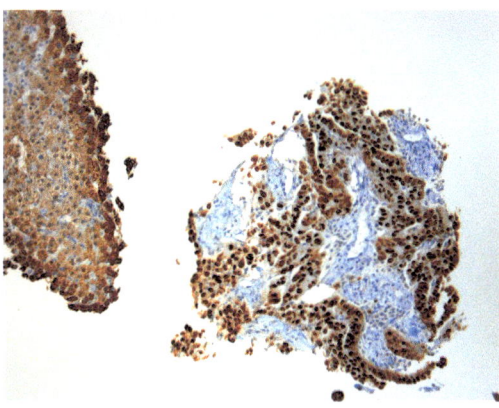

FɪG. 3.61.   Metastatic papillary thyroid carcinoma: A PAX-8 immunostain highlights the tumor cells (fragment on *right*) in this metastatic thyroid tumor in a patient with a known history. PAX-8 is a nuclear stain and also shows some intracytoplasmic granular positivity in the hepatocytes, which is of no significance. (PAX-8 immunostain, low power)

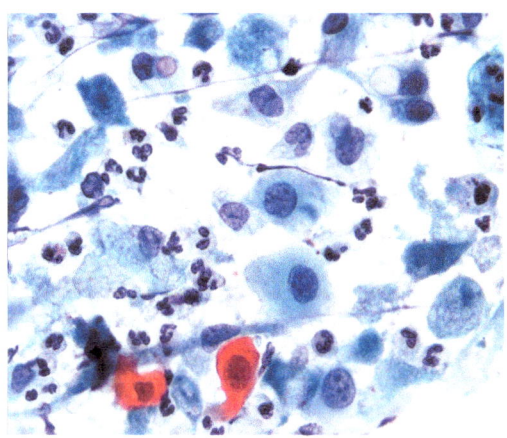

FɪG. 3.62.   Adenosquamous carcinoma, pancreatic primary: Clear evidence of squamous and glandular differentiation is shown in this image. There are cells with intracytoplasmic mucin vacuoles (2 o'clock) and others with keratinizing squamous differentiation (6 and 7 o'clock). The patient had a primary pancreatic adenosquamous carcinoma and multiple liver lesions. (Papanicolaou stain, high power)

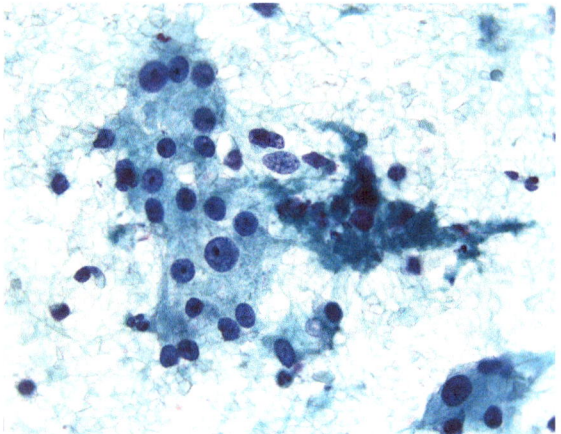

Fig. 3.63.   Metastatic Renal Cell carcinoma: A cohesive group of tumor cells is shown. The tumor cells have abundant vacuolated cytoplasm and ill-defined cell borders. The nuclei are round with single prominent nucleoli. A primary differential diagnostic consideration is hepatocellular carcinoma, though the cytoplasm is more vacuolated than granular. Immunostains might be required in the absence of a history of RCC. (Papanicolaou stain, medium power)

primary tumor, liver is one of the most common sites of metastasis for adrenal cortical carcinoma (ACC). The morphology bears some resemblance to HCC and thus consideration of ACC in the differential diagnosis is important. Morphologically, ACC shows polygonal cells, which are predominantly single on aspirate smears and show nuclear hyperchromasia with focal anisonucleosis. Nucleoli are not typically prominent, and there is no transgressing endothelium (Figs. 3.65, 3.66, and 3.67). Importantly, ACC may show endothelial cells enveloping small groups of hepatocytes on CB or NCB, thus immunostains may be necessary. ACCs express MelanA and inhibin and can express calretinin. They are negative for HepPar1 and pCEA.

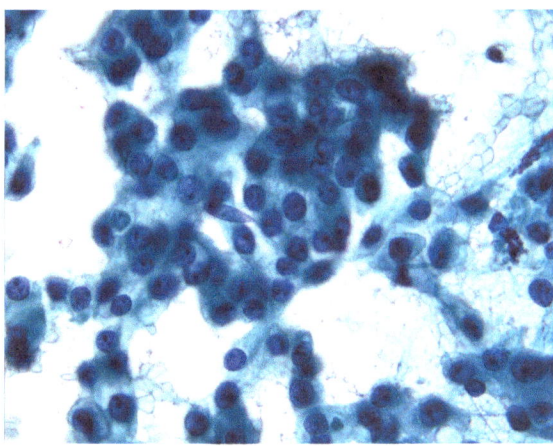

FIG. 3.64.   Metastatic Renal Cell carcinoma: Renal cell carcinoma is characteristically a vascular tumor and may show transgressing vessels, but not endothelial wrapping. A few small spindled cells are present in this image suggesting transgressing vessels admixed with the malignant epithelial cells. Cytoplasm is abundant and vacuolated and nucleoli are prominent. (Papanicolaou stain, high power)

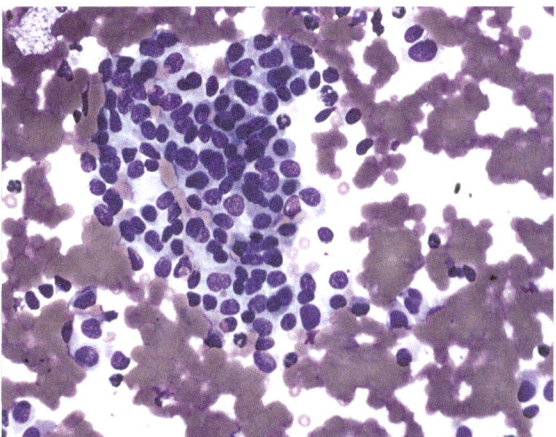

FIG. 3.65.   Metastatic Adrenal Cortical Carcinoma: These neoplastic cells show nuclear hyperchromasia and slight anisonucleosis. There is a moderate amount of cytoplasm, though less than what is seen in normal hepatocytes. The architecture is sheet like and does not show gland formation. (Diff-Quik stain, medium power)

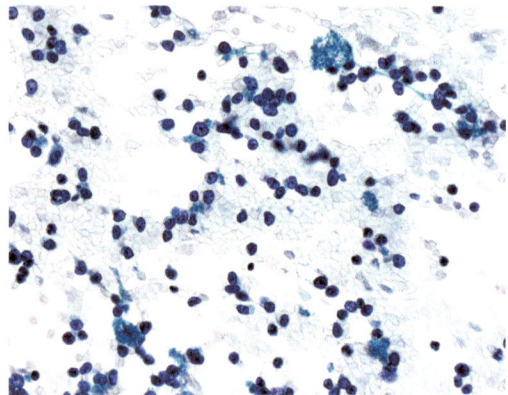

FIG. 3.66.   Metastatic Adrenal Cortical Carcinoma: The tumor cells present here are singly dispersed and show minimal anisonucleosis. The nuclei are hyperchromatic and there are small nucleoli. The differential diagnosis would include neuroendocrine tumors and malignant melanoma, but this patient had a history of adrenal cortical carcinoma. (Papanicolaou stain, medium power)

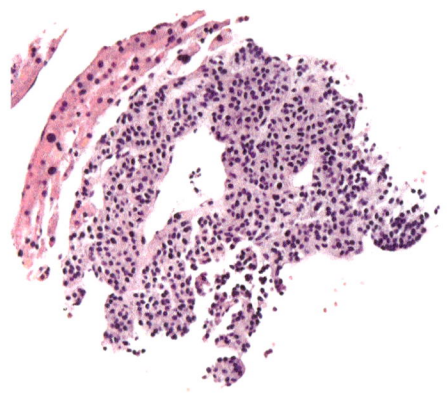

FIG. 3.67.   Metastatic Adrenal Cortical Carcinoma: This fragment of tissue present on the CB preparation shows tumor on the *right side* and a small amount of normal liver on the *left*. Small, spindled endothelial cells envelop groups of tumor cells, which is similar to the endothelial wrapping seen in HCC. This feature is not present on the aspirate smears in ACC, though. (Cell block, H&E stain, low power)

Suggested panel of immunostains for carcinoma (correlate with morphology and clinical history):

- HepPar1 (Hepatocellular carcinoma)
  - If positive proceed with reticulin, pCEA, CD34
- Ber-EP4 or MOC-31 (Most metastatic carcinomas)
  - If positive proceed with:

    CK7/CK20 (see Table 3.5)
    TTF-1
    CDX-2
    ER/PR
    PAX-8 (thyroid, kidney and GYN tract primary)

- If both negative, consider
  - S-100, MelanA, HMB-45
  - CD117 (C-Kit) (epithelioid GIST)

Metastatic Neuroendocrine Tumors

Primary hepatic neuroendocrine tumors are extremely rare, but are reported to occur. Common primary sites for metastatic neuroendocrine tumors in the liver include small bowel, pancreas, and liver, though neuroendocrine tumors from all sites show similar cytomorphology. Well-differentiated neuroendocrine tumors show characteristic features including a predominant population of monotonous single cells with associated small clusters of loosely cohesive cells. Nuclei are round and eccentrically placed (plasmacytoid) with finely dispersed chromatin. Nucleoli are unusual, though occasionally present. The cytoplasm is abundant and finely granular. Focal nuclear enlargement and atypia ("endocrine" atypia) may be present and do not indicate a higher grade lesion (Figs. 3.68, 3.69, and 3.70). Poorly differentiated neuroendocrine tumors (small cell carcinomas) are recognized by a population of cells with scant cytoplasm, neuroendocrine chromatin, and abundant mitotic figures as well as apoptotic debris. Nuclear molding and crush artifact are common (Figs. 3.71, 3.72, and 3.73). Immunohistochemical studies may

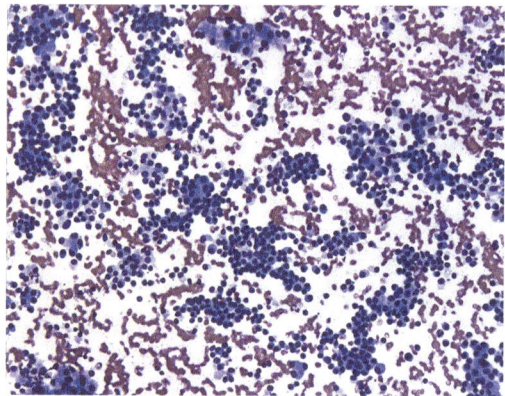

Fig. 3.68. Metastatic Well-differentiated neuroendocrine tumor: This very cellular aspirate shows a monotonous population of tumor cells in small aggregates and singly in the background. The nuclei are uniformly round and eccentrically placed. A small group of hepatocytes is present at 12 o'clock for comparison. The tumor cells are smaller overall and have slightly smaller nuclei than hepatocytes. (Diff-Quik stain, low power)

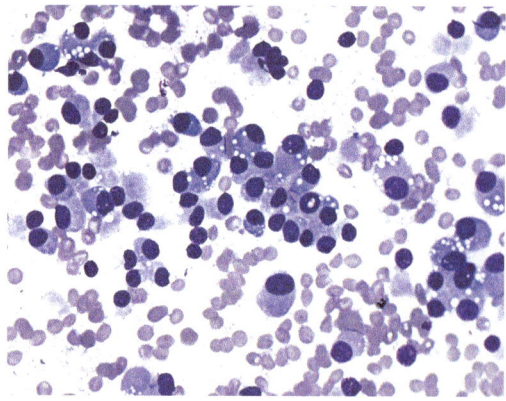

Fig. 3.69. Metastatic Well-differentiated neuroendocrine tumor: This is the typical appearance of a well-differentiated neuroendocrine tumor. The nuclei are uniformly round with smooth nuclear contours and are eccentrically placed within the cells. They are predominantly single cells with no distinct architectural pattern. (Diff-Quik stain, high power)

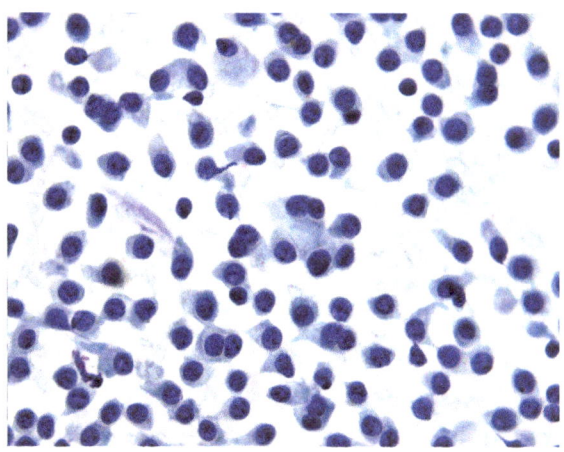

FIG. 3.70.   Metastatic Well-differentiated neuroendocrine tumor: These single tumor cells show the characteristic nuclear features of a neuroendocrine neoplasm. The chromatin is finely granular and there are no nucleoli. Nuclei are eccentrically placed within fairly abundant granular cytoplasm. (Papanicolaou stain, high power)

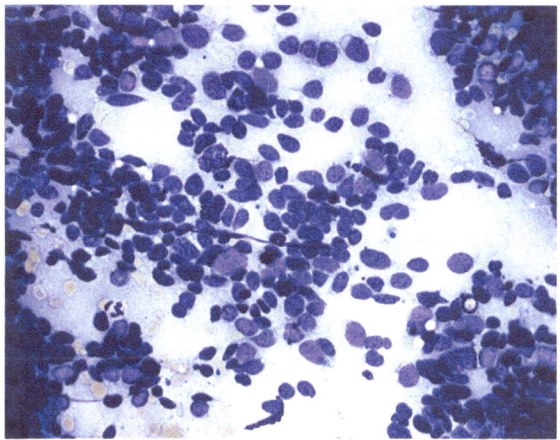

FIG. 3.71.   Metastatic Small cell carcinoma: This population of malignant cells shows large nuclei with very scant cytoplasm. Some nuclei show deformation by adjacent tumor nuclei known as "molding." Crushed tumor nuclei are also present in this image, which is characteristic of small cell carcinoma. (Diff-Quik stain, medium power)

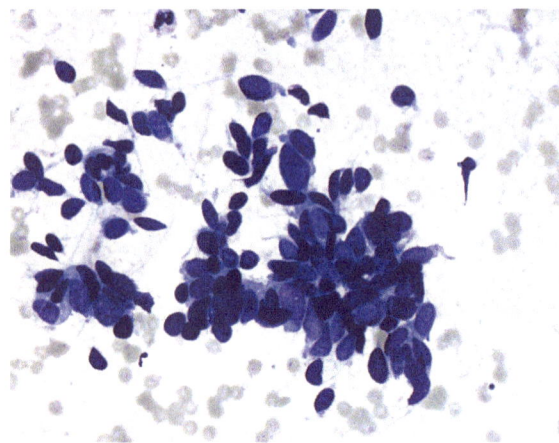

FIG. 3.72.   Metastatic Small cell carcinoma: These tumor cells have large, angulated nuclei with scant cytoplasm and display "molding." The finely dispersed chromatin is more difficult to appreciate on Diff Quik stain than Papanicolaou stain. (Diff-Quik stain, high power)

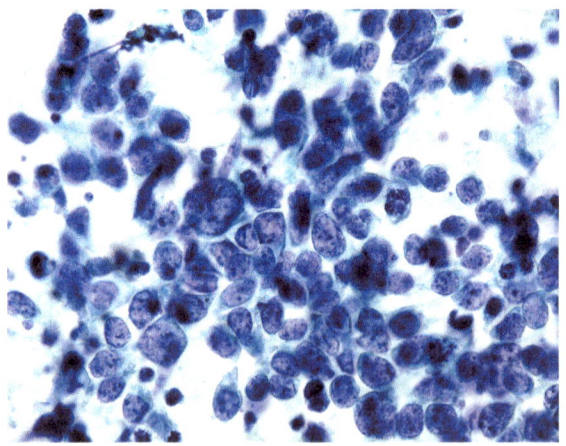

FIG. 3.73.   Metastatic Small cell carcinoma: The chromatin pattern in these malignant cells is typical of neuroendocrine origin. The nuclei are deformed and molded to one another. Mitotic figures and apoptotic debris are easily identified, as they should be in small cell carcinoma. (Papanicolaou stain, high power)

be performed on CB or NCB preparations. Neuroendocrine tumors are positive for Synaptophysin and Chromogranin A, typically strongly and diffusely. Ki67 mitotic index should be performed as it is important in the grading of these tumors. Small cell carcinoma from any site may be TTF-1 positive, thus it is not helpful in defining a primary site for a liver metastasis.

Key features:

- Combination of single cells and loosely cohesive clusters
- Monotonous cellular population with focal atypia
- Eccentric (plasmacytoid) nuclei
- Finely dispersed chromatin
- Granular cytoplasm
- High mitotic rate and apoptosis support small cell carcinoma

Differential diagnosis:

The differential diagnosis for a well-differentiated neuroendocrine tumor includes malignant melanoma (MM) (discussed below). Both may show a predominant single cell pattern with eccentric, round nuclei, but MMs typically have prominent nucleoli in contrast to the finely dispersed chromatin of neuroendocrine tumors. A poorly differentiated hepatocellular carcinoma or adenocarcinoma may be in the differential with small cell carcinoma, but the presence of nuclear molding and crush artifact, in conjunction with positive neuroendocrine immunostains, helps distinguish the tumors. Focal neuroendocrine differentiation can be seen in HCC and metastatic adenocarcinomas, but the staining should not be strong and diffuse as it is in neuroendocrine tumors.

Metastatic Malignant Melanoma

Metastatic malignant melanoma (MM) comprises 2.2 % of all liver metastases. Typically the patient has a known history, but metastases may result from an occult cutaneous or gastrointestinal primary. The cytomorphology of MM is famously varied as melanoma is known as the "great imitator."

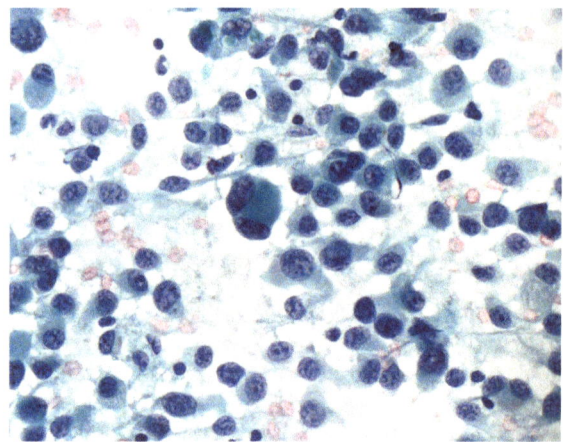

FIG. 3.74. Metastatic Malignant Melanoma: Though malignant melanoma can show widely varied morphologic appearances, this is a typical appearance for the neoplasm. Cells are arranged singly and show round to slightly oval shaped nuclei which are eccentrically placed in abundant cytoplasm. The nucleoli here are not as prominent as typically seen in MM. A binucleated cell is present in the *center* of the field. (Papanicolaou stain, medium power)

Classically, aspirate smears show predominantly single monotonous tumor cells with occasional marked nuclear enlargement. Nuclei are eccentrically placed (plasmacytoid) and binucleation is common. Nucleoli are usually very prominent and intranuclear inclusions are often present. Melanin pigment may be present. MMs are immunoreactive for S-100 (most sensitive), MelanA, and HMB-45 (Figs. 3.74, 3.75, and 3.76).

Key features:

- Single, uniform cells
- Occasional pleomorphism and marked nuclear enlargement
- Eccentric (plasmacytoid) nuclei
- Binucleation
- Prominent nucleoli

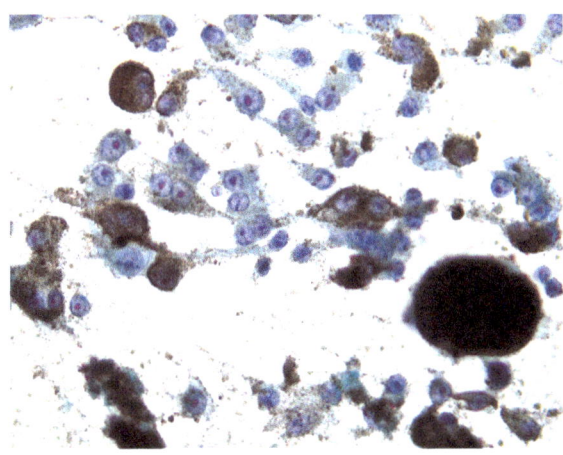

FIG. 3.75.   Metastatic Malignant Melanoma: These malignant cells show relatively uniformly sized, round nuclei with prominent *cherry-red* nucleoli. There is abundant cytoplasm and dense melanin pigment is present in many cells, which makes the diagnosis straightforward. (Papanicolaou stain, medium power)

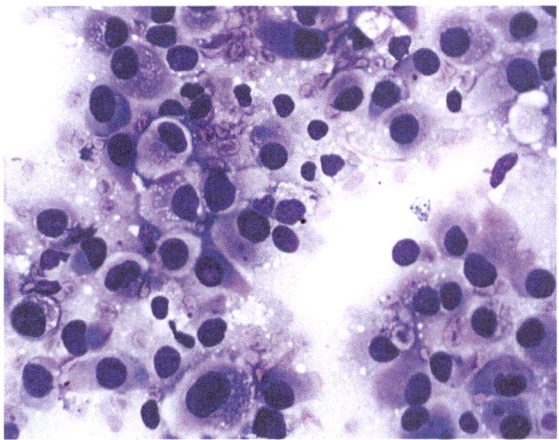

FIG. 3.76.   Metastatic Malignant Melanoma: These tumor cells are singly dispersed and show round to oval nuclei with abundant granular cytoplasm. An intranuclear inclusion is present at approximately 7 o'clock, which is common in MM. The differential diagnosis in this case would include HCC. (Diff-Quik stain, high power)

- Intranuclear inclusions
- Granular cytoplasm
- Melanin pigment

Differential diagnosis:
As MM is the "great imitator," it can resemble many other tumors. The classical presentation of MM as singly dispersed cells with eccentric nuclei raises the differential of a neuroendocrine tumor. The prominent nucleoli seen in MM are distinctly uncommon in neuroendocrine tumors. Metastatic carcinomas of any type may resemble MM if the MM forms clusters that appear epithelioid. In particular, HCC may be in the differential given prominent nucleoli and granular cytoplasm. Immunostains for melanoma markers and keratins (negative in MM) are useful. Melanomas are negative for HepPar1 and pCEA

Metastatic Spindle Cell Neoplasms

Any sarcoma or spindle cell neoplasm can metastasize to liver. Metastatic sarcomas are more common than primary hepatic sarcoma, so clinical history, including physical exam and radiographic findings, is important in assessing sarcomas in the liver. Immunohistochemistry can be helpful in definitively diagnosing some spindle cell neoplasms, but some sarcomas, such as undifferentiated pleomorphic sarcoma, do not have a specific immunostaining profile that can confirm the diagnosis. Leiomyosarcomas and GISTs are the most common primary sarcomas to metastasize to liver.

Cytomorphologically, GISTs show cohesive groups of monomorphic spindle cells often with small blood vessels traversing the fragments. Individual cells show bland nuclei with delicate cytoplasmic processes. Paranuclear vacuoles may be present. Focal eosinophilic or myxoid stroma may be present in the background of aspirate smears or may be admixed with the spindle cell component. The epithelioid variant of GIST may be difficult to distinguish from carcinoma or a neuroendocrine tumor. Immunohistochemical studies for CK117 (C-Kit) and CD34 are positive in the conventional and epithelioid types of GIST and very useful in confirming the diagnosis. Aspirate smears from leiomyosarcoma show a population of pleomorphic spindle cells arranged in cohesive groups with scattered single cells in the background. The nuclei vary in size and shape depending on the grade of tumor, and have wiry cytoplasmic processes. Immunohistochemical stains for Desmin and smooth muscle actin are positive. Other sarcomas are recognized by their spindle-shaped nuclei with varying degrees of pleomorphism and a background stroma or matrix, which may be present.

Differential diagnosis:
Distinguishing a primary from a metastatic spindle cell neoplasm in the liver may not be possible without correlation with clinical and radiographic findings as they are morphologically identical. Malignant melanoma may show a spindled morphology, but typically shows more epithelioid nuclei and prominent nucleoli, which are uncommon in sarcomas. Tumor cells in melanoma are more often dispersed singly, and immunostains for melanoma are helpful. Epithelioid GIST can be mistaken for an epithelial neoplasm, but immunostains for CD117 and CD34 (positive) as well as keratins (negative) are helpful in the diagnosis.

Metastatic Hematopoietic Neoplasms

Lymphomas involving the liver generally involve the portal tracts and form nodular masses. Large-cell lymphomas, particularly diffuse large B-cell lymphomas, are the most common lymphomas to involve liver (Figs. 3.77 and 3.78). Small cell lymphoma (follicular lymphoma, mucosa-associated lymphoma tissue (MALT) lymphoma, and small lymphocytic lymphoma) are less common, and a clinical history of the disease is helpful to aid in recognition and triage of the specimen for flow cytometry. Peripheral T-cell lymphomas, though uncommon overall, involve liver in up to 50 % of cases. Hodgkin lymphoma involves the liver, typically as a secondary or metastatic site, and forms nodular masses in the portal tracts (Fig. 3.79). Leukemia involves the liver in a diffuse sinusoidal pattern, except CLL and ALL which often involve portal tracts.

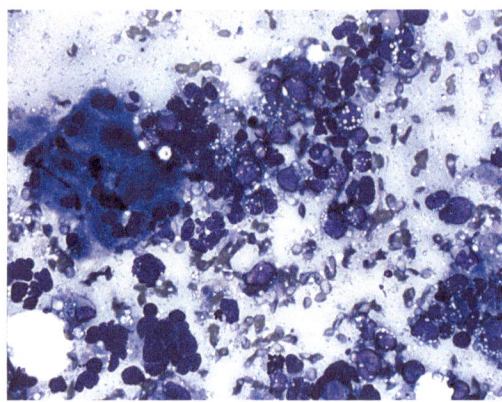

FIG. 3.77.   Metastatic Diffuse Large B-cell lymphoma: The neoplastic cells shown here are singly dispersed and show a very high nuclear to cytoplasmic ratio. The scant cytoplasm is *deep blue* on Diff Quik stain, characteristic of lymphoid cells. A group of hepatocytes is present in the *upper left* for reference. (Diff-Quik stain, medium power)

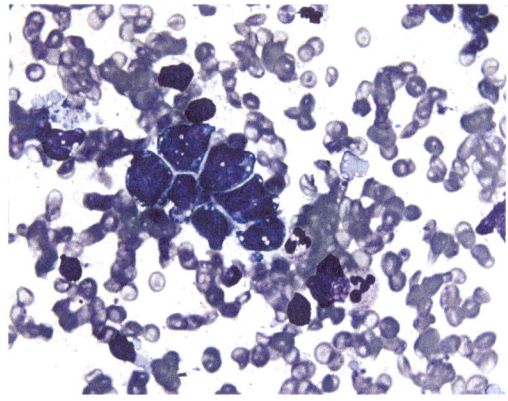

FIG. 3.78.   Metastatic Diffuse Large B-cell lymphoma: On high magnification, malignant cells with very high nuclear to cytoplasmic ratios, irregular nuclear contours, and scant *deep blue* cytoplasm are seen, consistent with a large B-cell lymphoma. In air dried smears, focal areas similar to small cell carcinoma may be seen. Flow cytometry studies are very useful in this setting to confirm that a clonal population of lymphoid cells is present. (Diff-Quik stain, high power)

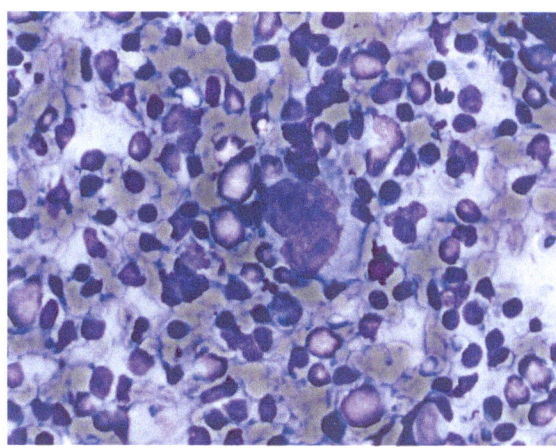

Fig. 3.79. Metastatic Hodgkin Lymphoma: A very large Reed-Sternberg cell is present in the *center* of the image showing binucleation and prominent nucleoli. The background shows a mixed inflammatory infiltrate, predominantly lymphocytes and few plasma cells. In a patient with a history of HL, these findings are consistent with liver involvement. For a primary diagnosis of HL, core biopsies and immunostains are needed. (Diff-Quik stain, high power)

Cytomorphology of lymphoma and leukemia is identical to those diagnoses made at other sites. Generally, hematopoietic neoplasms show single, dispersed cells with small rims of blue cytoplasm on Diff-Quik staining, which is the preferred stain to evaluate these neoplasms. Small fragments of cytoplasm known as lymphoglandular bodies are found scattered in the background (Diff-Quik stain). Flow cytometry and clinical history are important to make the diagnosis. Large cell lymphomas show markedly enlarged lymphocytes with irregular nuclear membranes and may have prominent nucleoli. Small cell lymphoma is composed of a population of monotonous small to moderate-sized lymphocytes, which are difficult to distinguish from normal lymphocytes on morphology, though the presence of large aggregates of lymphocytes in the liver is atypical. On close examination, the lymphocytes may have irregular nuclear contours, clefts, and nucleoli, which are not typically seen in benign lymphocytes.

TABLE 3.6. Immunohistochemical profile of neoplasms commonly metastatic to liver.

Primary tumor	Positive immunostains
Breast carcinoma	ER, PR, GCDFP15, Mammoglobin
Ovarian serous carcinoma	WT1, CA125, PAX8
Prostate carcinoma	PSA, PSMA, p501s
Urothelial carcinoma	p63, GATA3
Colon carcinoma	CDX2, CK20
Pancreas and biliary tree	Loss of DPC4, CK19
Lung adenocarcinoma	TTF-1, Napsin A
Lung small cell carcinoma, any site	TTF-1
Endometrial carcinoma	ER, PR
Renal cell carcinoma	PAX8, vimentin, RCCma, CD10
Adrenal cortical carcinoma	Inhibin, Melan A
Thyroid (papillary or follicular carcinoma)	TTF1, Thyroglobulin, PAX8
Neuroendocrine tumor	Synaptophysin, Chromogranin A
Malignant Melanoma	S-100, Melan A, HMB-45, SOX-10, MITF
Gastrointestinal Stromal Tumor	C-kit (CD117), CD34
Non-Hodgkin lymphoma	CD45 (LCA), CD3, CD20 (depending on type)
Hodgkin lymphoma	CD30, CD15

Flow cytometry studies and immunohistochemical stains showing positivity for CD45 (leukocyte common antigen) and other B- and T-cell markers including CD3 and CD20 are helpful.

Differential diagnosis:

Lymphomas and leukemias are typically recognized by their dispersed, single cell arrangement and the distinct deep blue cytoplasmic rim, but on occasion a high grade large cell lymphoma may resemble a poorly differentiated carcinoma. Hematopoietic cells can give the appearance of forming aggregates if allowed to clot during fine needle aspiration allowing overlap with a carcinoma diagnosis. Flow cytometry and immunohistochemical studies readily differentiate the two.

As virtually any neoplasm may involve the liver, immunostaining is often needed to distinguish the primary site. A general reference table is provided above (Table 3.6).

Suggested Reading

Contraindications

Assy N, Nasser G, Djibre A, et al. Characteristics of common solid liver lesions and recommendations for diagnostic workup. World J Gastroenterol. 2009a;15:3217–27.

Bravo AA, Sheth SG, Chopra S. Liver biopsy. N Engl J Med. 2001;344:495–500.

Franca AV, Valerio HM, Trevisan M, et al. Fine needle aspiration biopsy for improving the diagnostic accuracy of cut needle biopsy of focal liver lesions. Acta Cytol. 2003;47:332–6.

Grant A, Neuberger J. Guidelines on the use of liver biopsy in clinical practice. British Society of Gastroenterology. Gut. 1999;45 Suppl 4:IV1–11.

Karhunen PJ. Benign hepatic tumours and tumour like conditions in men. J Clin Pathol. 1986;39:183–8.

McGill DB, Rakela J, Zinsmeister AR, et al. A 21-year experience with major hemorrhage after percutaneous liver biopsy. Gastroenterology. 1990;99:1396–400.

Schwartz LH, Gandras EJ, Colangelo SM, et al. Prevalence and importance of small hepatic lesions found at CT in patients with cancer. Radiology. 1999;210:71–4.

Stewart CJ, Coldewey J, Stewart IS. Comparison of fine needle aspiration cytology and needle core biopsy in the diagnosis of radiologically detected abdominal lesions. J Clin Pathol. 2002;55:93–7.

Winter TC, Lee Jr FT, Hinshaw JL. Ultrasound-guided biopsies in the abdomen and pelvis. Ultrasound Q. 2008;24:45–68.

Pigments

Guy CD, Ballo MS. Fine needle aspiration biopsy of the liver. Adv Anat Pathol. 1999;6:303–16.

Hepatobiliary Cystadenoma

Ahmad I, Iyer A, Marginean CE, et al. Diagnostic use of cytokeratins, CD34, and neuronal cell adhesion molecule staining in focal nodular hyperplasia and hepatic adenoma. Hum Pathol. 2009; 40:726–34.

Cohen MB, Haber MM, Holly EA, et al. Cytologic criteria to distinguish hepatocellular carcinoma from nonneoplastic liver. Am J Clin Pathol. 1991;95:125–30.

Hussain SM, Terkivatan T, Zondervan PE, et al. Focal nodular hyperplasia: findings at state-of-the-art MR imaging, US, CT, and pathologic analysis. Radiographics. 2004;24:3–19.

Parwani AV, Burroughs FH, Ali SZ. Echinococcal cyst of the liver. Diagn Cytopathol. 2004;31:111–2.

Ruschenburg I, Droese M. Fine needle aspiration cytology of focal nodular hyperplasia of the liver. Acta Cytol. 1989;33:857–60.

Yang GC, Yang GY, Tao LC. Distinguishing well-differentiated hepatocellular carcinoma from benign liver by the physical features of fine-needle aspirates. Mod Pathol. 2004;17:798–802.

Rare Primary Malignant Neoplasms

Assy N, Nasser G, Djibre A, et al. Characteristics of common solid liver lesions and recommendations for diagnostic workup. World J Gastroenterol. 2009b;15:3217–27.

Barwad A, Gupta N, Gupta K, et al. Hepatoblastoma—an attempt of histological subtyping on fine-needle aspiration material. Diagn Cytopathol. 2013;41:95–101.

Das DK. Cytodiagnosis of hepatocellular carcinoma in fine-needle aspirates of the liver: its differentiation from reactive hepatocytes and metastatic adenocarcinoma. Diagn Cytopathol. 1999;21: 370–7.

Kakar S, Gown AM, Goodman ZD, et al. Best practices in diagnostic immuno-histochemistry: hepatocellular carcinoma versus metastatic neoplasms. Arch Pathol Lab Med. 2007a;131:1648–54.

Kulesza P, Torbenson M, Sheth S, et al. Cytopathologic grading of hepatocellular carcinoma on fine-needle aspiration. Cancer. 2004;102:247–58.

Wakely Jr PE, Silverman JF, Geisinger KR, et al. Fine needle aspiration biopsy cytology of hepatoblastoma. Mod Pathol. 1990;3: 688–93.

Wee A. Fine needle aspiration biopsy of hepatocellular carcinoma and hepatocellular nodular lesions: role, controversies and approach to diagnosis. Cytopathology. 2001;220:287–305.

Metastatic Neoplasms to Liver

Centeno BA. Pathology of liver metastases. Cancer Control. 2006; 13:13–26.

Kakar S, Gown AM, Goodman ZD, et al. Best practices in diagnostic immunohistochemistry: hepatocellular carcinoma versus meta-static neoplasms. Arch Pathol Lab Med. 2007b;131:1648–54.

Chapter 4
Biliary Tract

Specimen Procurement and Preparation

Brush sampling of the bile ducts is performed either during endoscopic retrograde cholangiopancreatography (ERCP) or aspirated during percutaneous transhepatic cholangiography. Brushes can be directly smeared onto slides and stained using either Diff-Quik or Papanicolaou stain. They are either submitted intact submerged in ethanol-based solution, prepared by Cytospin method, and stained with Papanicolaou stain, or rinsed in a liquid-based cytology preservative solution and prepared using the liquid-based cytology platform methods. Some studies report improved detection of adenocarcinoma in bile duct brushings prepared using ThinPrep® technology over conventional smears due to better cellular preservation. There are no standardized criteria for adequacy in bile duct brushings or aspirations.

The reported sensitivity ranges from 30 to 88 % (mean 55 %). This relatively low sensitivity is attributed to either sampling error or interpretative error. Sampling error may be due to lesion size, location, extensive fibrosis, benign epithelium overlying a mass lesion, or technical difficulties, possibly related to experience of operator. Interpretative errors result from subtle changes in well-differentiated neoplasms which are difficult to definitively diagnose, or from

Y.S. Erozan and A. Tatsas, *Cytopathology of Liver,*
Biliary Tract, Kidney and Adrenal Gland, Essentials
in Cytopathology 18, DOI 10.1007/978-1-4899-7513-3_4,
© Springer Science+Business Media New York 2015

lack of familiarity with the specimen type and poor cellular preservation. Sensitivity can be increased with repeat brushing. The overall reported specificity is 87–100 % (mean 97 %), thus the diagnosis is quite reliable if positive for malignancy.

Benign/Normal Biliary Epithelium

It is important to recognize the features of benign and reactive biliary epithelium in order to accurately diagnose adenocarcinoma in bile duct specimens. Benign biliary epithelium displays an orderly flat sheet of evenly spaced nuclei displaying a "honeycomb" arrangement. The nuclei are uniform in size, round to oval, with smooth nuclear contours and little to no nuclear overlap, and they are typically centrally placed in the cytoplasm of the cell. The nuclear to cytoplasmic ratio is low, though not as low as hepatocytes, as there is a moderate amount of finely granular cytoplasm, in contrast to the coarsely granular cytoplasm of hepatocytes. Small nucleoli are acceptable in benign epithelium (Figs. 4.1 and 4.2).

Key features:

- Cohesive orderly monolayer sheets with a "honeycomb" arrangement
- Evenly spaced, uniformly sized nuclei
- Little to no nuclear overlap
- Moderate amount of finely granular cytoplasm
- Low n/c ratio
- Round to oval nuclei with smooth nuclear contours
- Occasional small nucleoli

Reactive Biliary Epithelium

Reactive epithelium may result from bouts of chronic pancreatitis, stones, or stent placement and can show focal marked atypia that may be mistaken for adenocarcinoma.

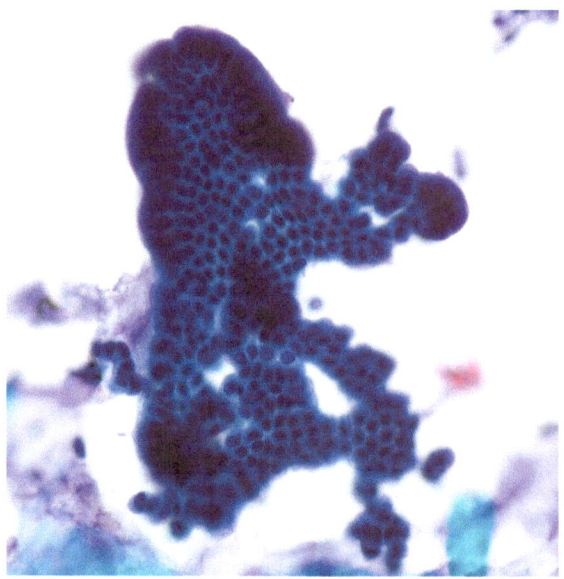

FIG. 4.1. Biliary epithelium, normal: A fragment of normal, well-organized biliary epithelium is shown. The nuclei are small and evenly spaced in a honey comb arrangement with no overlap. (Biliary duct brush, Papanicolaou stain, medium power)

Disruption of the normal "honeycomb" architecture occurs with unevenly spaced nuclei. Nuclei are often enlarged, typically in the range of two to three times normal size, and show small- to intermediate-sized nucleoli, sometimes multiple. Importantly, nuclear contours are smooth in contrast to the nuclear membrane irregularities seen in adenocarcinoma. The background in reactive processes often shows inflammatory cells, acute or chronic, and may show debris and bile pigment. If inflammatory cells are embedded in the ductal epithelium, a diagnosis of reactive atypia should be strongly considered prior to rendering a malignant diagnosis (Figs. 4.3, 4.4, 4.5, and 4.6).

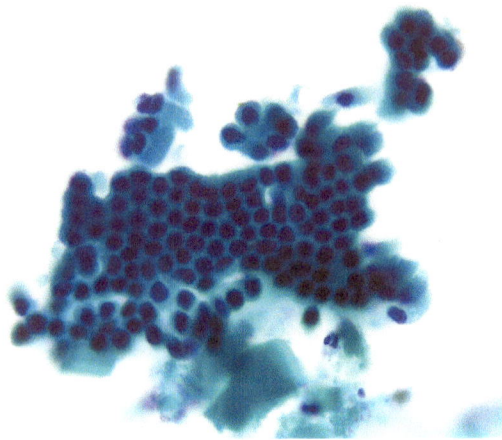

FIG. 4.2.   Biliary epithelium, normal: This fragment of biliary epithelium shows evenly sized, round nuclei which are centrally placed in a moderate amount of cytoplasm with ill-defined cell borders. The nuclei are uniformly spaced and show no overlap. (Biliary duct brush, Papanicolaou stain, medium power)

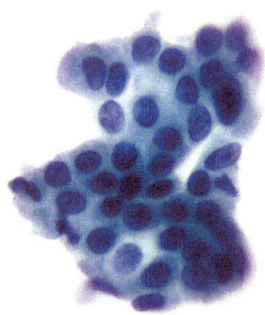

FIG. 4.3.   Biliary epithelium, reactive: This fragment of biliary epithelium shows very mild nuclear enlargement and slight disorganization of the honeycomb arrangement, though there is still no nuclear overlap. Nuclear contours are smooth and there are scattered small nucleoli. (Biliary duct brush, Papanicolaou stain, high power)

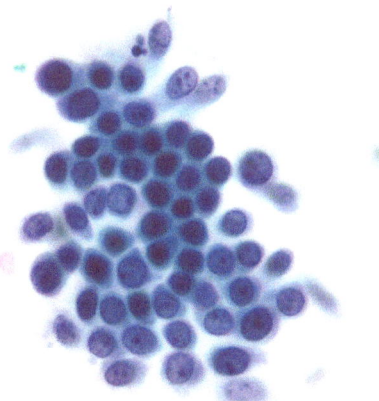

FIG. 4.4.   Biliary epithelium, reactive: Slight nuclear hyperchromasia and enlargement are shown, characteristic of a benign reactive process. Small nucleoli are easily identified, but the nuclear contours are still very smooth, in contrast to what is seen in neoplastic processes. (Biliary duct brush, Papanicolaou stain, high power)

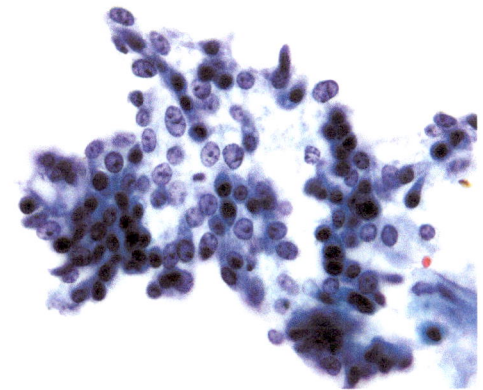

FIG. 4.5.   Biliary epithelium, reactive: The architecture in this fragment of biliary epithelium is quite disorganized and the nuclei are enlarged, though only two to three times normal. Nucleoli are present in most cells and the chromatin distribution is somewhat irregular. This patient had a history of primary biliary cirrhosis and had a series of reactive biliary brushings. (Biliary duct brush, Papanicolaou stain, medium power)

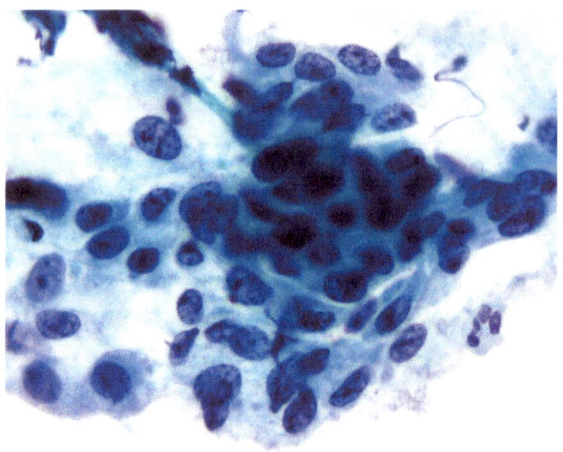

FIG. 4.6.   Biliary epithelium, reactive: This epithelium is quite reactive and is from a patient who had a stent in place prior to the brushing. The nuclei are enlarged and have moderate size nucleoli. The nuclear contours are smooth and the nuclear enlargement is only in the two to three times range, favoring a reactive process. A degenerated neutrophil is seen at 4 o'clock, which also supports a reactive process. (Biliary duct brush, Papanicolaou stain, high power)

Key features:

- Mild architectural disruption with focally uneven nuclear spacing, but little overlap
- Slight nuclear enlargement (two to three times normal)
- Small- to intermediate-sized nucleoli, sometimes multiple
- Smooth nuclear contours
- Embedded or background inflammatory cells

Infectious Organisms

Liver flukes such as *Clonorchis sinensis* (*Opisthorchis sinensis*) and *Opisthorchis viverrini* infect the biliary tract. These infections are quite uncommon in the United States, but are prevalent in Southeast Asia. The infections are rarely

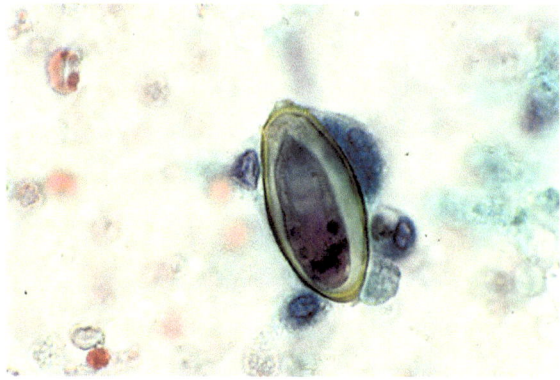

FIG. 4.7. *Clonorchis sinensis* ovum: A small, oval shaped egg from a *Clonorchis sinensis* infection of the biliary tree is shown. (Biliary duct brush, Papanicolaou stain, high power)

symptomatic and may persist for decades. Prolonged infection may cause cholangitis and pancreatitis and place patients at increased risk for cholangiocarcinoma. Rarely, the ova may be seen on a biliary brush specimen (Fig. 4.7).

Cholangiocarcinoma

Cholangiocarcinoma represents 10–15 % of hepatobiliary malignancies. Risk factors include parasitic infection (Clonorchis sinensis, Opisthorchis viverrini), primary sclerosing cholangitis (PSC), primary biliary cirrhosis, Choledochal cysts, Caroli syndrome, cholelithiasis, Thorotrast exposure, and chronic liver disease. Primary sclerosing cholangitis is the most important causative factor in the Western world, and 6–36 % of patients with PSC develop cholangiocarcinoma. These patients are monitored by serial ERCP-directed bile duct brushings. The lesions are most often hilar (40–60 %), followed by extrahepatic (20–30 %), and peripheral (10–15 %). The extrahepatic tumors involve distal common bile duct, and patients present with painless jaundice.

Imaging shows dilated intrahepatic bile ducts. Three-year survival rates for resectable tumors are around 50 %.

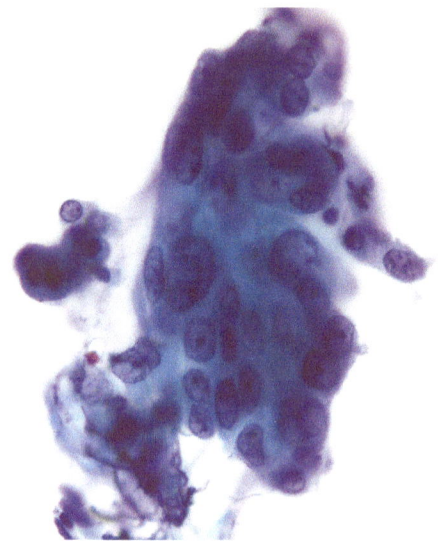

FIG. 4.8. Cholangiocarcinoma: This fragment shows the marked atypia characteristic of adenocarcinoma. A small group of benign biliary cells is present at 9 o'clock and, in contrast, the group of cells on the *right* shows nuclear enlargement more than four times a normal nucleus as well as nuclear contour irregularities and prominent nucleoli. (Biliary duct brush, Papanicolaou stain, high power)

Metastases are usually to lymph nodes, lung, liver, and peritoneal cavity.

The cytopathologic features of cholangiocarcinoma are similar to those seen in other adenocarcinomas. The normal honeycomb architecture of bile duct epithelium is completely disrupted, and there is nuclear crowding and overlap. Anisonucleosis is significant, and nuclear enlargement greater than four times normal size should be present. The nuclear to cytoplasmic ratio is thus increased with the increased nuclear size. Nuclear contours are irregular, notched, and jagged, and chromatin becomes coarse and clumped. Nucleoli may be absent to prominent. The presence of scattered single malignant cells in the background of preparations is also very common, though not necessary for the diagnosis (Figs. 4.8, 4.9, 4.10, and 4.11).

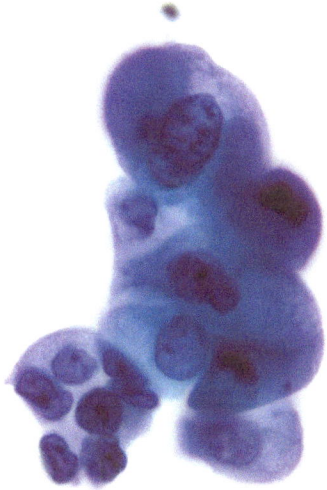

FIG. 4.9.   Cholangiocarcinoma: These malignant cells have mark-edly enlarged nuclei with irregular shapes and notched nuclear membranes. Chromatin is irregularly distributed and there are small nucleoli. Architectural organization is completely lost. (Biliary duct brush, Papanicolaou stain, high power)

Key features:

- Tissue fragments with marked disorganization of honey-comb architecture
- Scattered single malignant cells
- Marked anisonucleosis
- Nuclear enlargement (greater than four times normal)
- Increased n/c ratio
- Irregular nuclear contours
- Coarse, clumped chromatin
- Variably prominent nucleoli

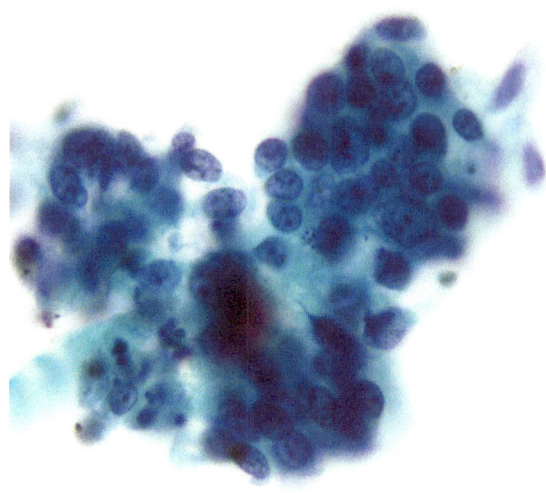

FIG. 4.10.   Cholangiocarcinoma: This tissue fragment of tumor cells shows disorganization including nuclear overlap and crowding. Nuclei are enlarged, irregularly shaped and have jagged nuclear contours. Nucleoli are moderate in size. (Biliary duct brush, Papanicolaou stain, high power)

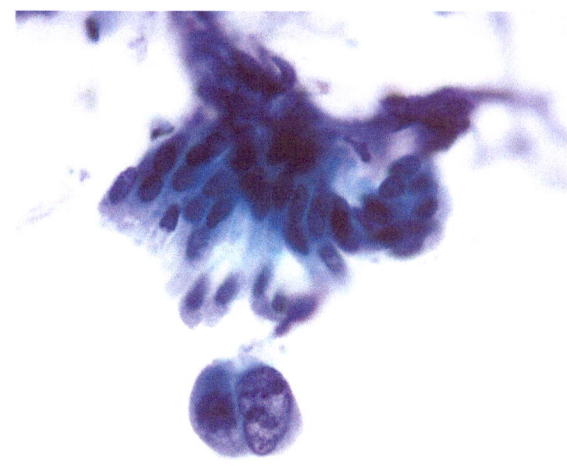

Fɪɢ. 4.11.   Cholangiocarcinoma: An enormous single tumor cell is present at 6 o'clock in this image. The nuclear to cytoplasmic ratio is high and the nuclear contours are very irregular. Some benign biliary epithelium is shown at the *top* of the image for reference. Single malignant cells are very helpful in making the diagnosis of adenocarcinoma in a brushing sample. (Biliary duct brush, Papanicolaou stain, high power)

Suggested Reading

Cohen MB, Wittchow R, Johlin FC, et al. Brush cytology of the extrahepatic biliary tract: comparison of cytologic features of adenocarcinoma and benign biliary strictures. Mod Pathol. 1995;8: 498–502.

Curley SA. Biliary tract cancer. Cancer Treat Res. 1997;90:273–307.

Henke AC, Jensen CS, Cohen MB. Cytologic diagnosis of adenocarcinoma in biliary and pancreatic duct brushings. Adv Anat Pathol. 2002;9:301–8.

Jarnagin WR. Cholangiocarcinoma of the extrahepatic bile ducts. Semin Surg Oncol. 2000;19:156–76.

Selvaggi SM. Biliary brushing cytology. Cytopathology. 2004;15: 74–9.

Siddiqui MT, Gokaslan ST, Saboorian MH, et al. Comparison of ThinPrep and conventional smears in detecting carcinoma in bile duct brushings. Cancer. 2003;99:205–10.

Chapter 5
Kidney

Introduction

Computed tomography (CT)- or ultrasound (US)-guided fine needle aspirations (FNAs) and core biopsies (CB) are increasingly used for the diagnosis of mass lesions of kidney detected by imaging techniques. Although clinical and radiological findings would be adequate to determine the benign or malignant nature of the lesion in most cases, in some, ruling out a metastatic neoplasm or a more specific diagnosis of the type of tumor may be needed to choose the appropriate therapy (e.g., total vs partial nephrectomy, cryoablation, neoadjuvant-targeted therapy).

FNAs have been used alone or in combination with core biopsies. Multiple regions of a large tumor can be sampled by FNA with lesser risk of complications, and it could also help to direct the core biopsy to the site which is best representative of the lesion if done in combination with core biopsies.

Normal Components

Varying numbers of renal tubules and glomeruli may be found in fine needle aspirations. Glomeruli appear as thick, rounded structures with dense centers (Fig. 5.1).

Y.S. Erozan and A. Tatsas, *Cytopathology of Liver, Biliary Tract, Kidney and Adrenal Gland*, Essentials in Cytopathology 18, DOI 10.1007/978-1-4899-7513-3_5, © Springer Science+Business Media New York 2015

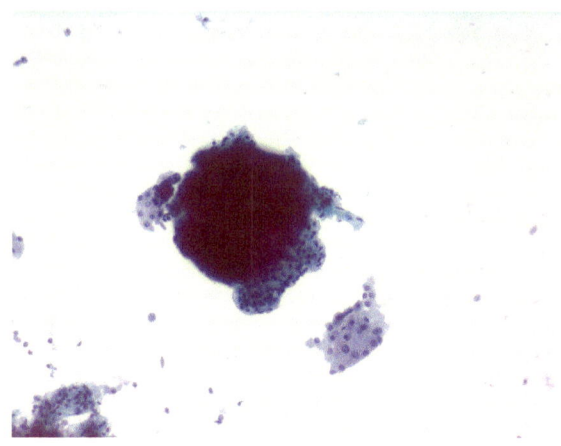

FIG. 5.1.   Glomerulus: Note fragment of proximal tubular epithelium. (Papanicolaou stain, medium power)

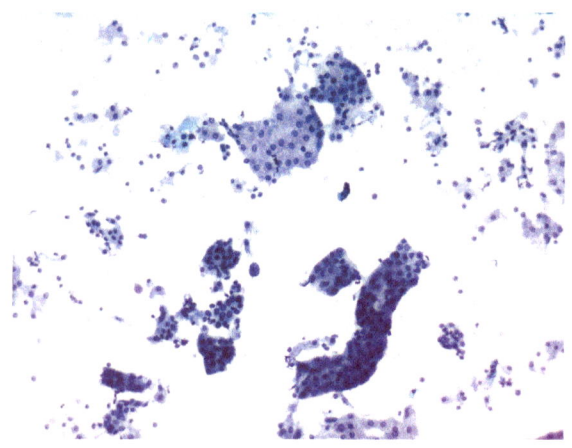

FIG. 5.2.   Renal tubular epithelium. (Papanicolaou stain, low power)

Renal tubules are seen as small monolayer tissue fragments,
groups, or tubular structures (Figs. 5.2 and 5.3). They may be
mistaken for well-differentiated renal cell carcinoma in limited specimens.

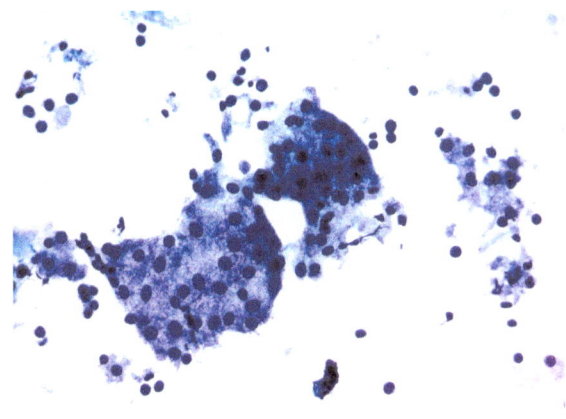

FIG. 5.3.   Fragment of proximal tubular epithelium: (Papanicolaou stain, medium power)

Nonneoplastic Masses and Cystic Lesions

Xanthogranulomatous Pyelonephritis (XGP)

Xanthogranulomatous pyelonephritis is a chronic inflammatory disease of kidney predominantly occurring in women. In 90 % of these cases, the kidney is diffusely involved. In a small percentage of cases, XGP is focal, forming a mass lesion mimicking renal cell carcinoma. Histologically it is composed of lipid-laden macrophages mixed with lymphocytes and plasma cells. Lipid-laden macrophages may mimic the clear cells of the conventional RCC.

Cytomorphology:
Misdiagnosis of XGP as renal cell carcinoma has been reported in FNAs and urine specimens. In FNA specimens, lipid-laden macrophages with vacuolated cytoplasm and vesicular nuclei with prominent nucleoli may mimic clear cell RCC. The cases showing an inflammatory background with predominantly lymphocytes, plasma cells, and occasional multinucleated cells mixed with histiocytes can be diagnosed as or suspected of being XPG in FNA specimens (Fig. 5.4a–c).

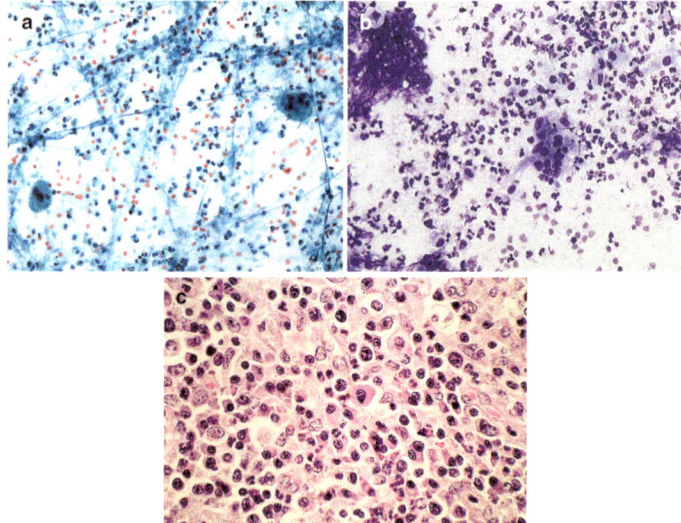

FIG. 5.4. Xanthogranulomatous pyelonephritis: Multinucleated giant cells in a background of lymphocytes, neutrophils, and macrophages. (**a**) (Papanicolaou stain, low power). (**b**) (Diff-Quik stain, medium power). (**c**) Predominantly mononuclear cells, some with significant nuclear atypia (Cell block, H&E stain, medium power)

Key features:

- Varying number of lipid-laden macrophages
- Lymphocytic/plasmocytic background

Differential diagnosis:

Conventional (clear cell) RCC is the main tumor to be considered in the differential diagnosis. In cases with predominantly lipid-laden macrophages, CD68 stain on cell blocks or core biopsies confirm the diagnosis of XPG.

Abscess

Retroperitoneal abscesses in the kidney region are usually secondary to bacterial infection at another location. They can be confined to the kidney, occur in the perirenal region, or

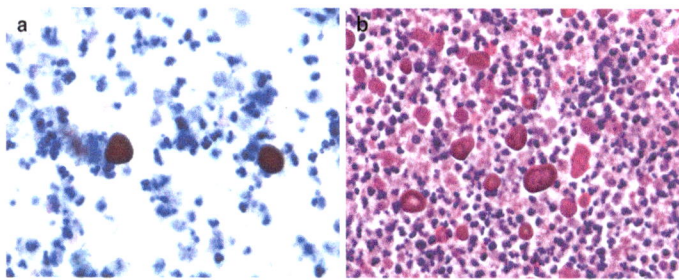

FIG. 5.5.   Renal cyst: Liesegang rings in a background of macrophages. (**a**) (Papanicolaou stain, medium power). (**b**) (Cell block, H&E stain, medium power)

mixed. Abscesses confined to the renal parenchyma are rare and can be treated medically. Others usually require drainage or more invasive surgical procedures.

In aspiration specimens, neutrophils are the predominant cell component. In addition, rare degenerated renal tubular cells and macrophages may be present.

Benign Cysts

Benign renal cysts are common findings in older individuals. They are usually unilocular and are diagnosed radiologically. There are, however, some benign cysts which have atypical imaging and cytological features which make the differential diagnosis from malignant neoplasms difficult.

Aspiration specimens of benign cysts usually contain predominantly macrophages. Fragments of cyst lining epithelium and renal tubular epithelium could be present. Rarely, round lamellated structures (Liesegang rings) are present (Fig. 5.5a, b). In rare cases, histiocytes or epithelial lining cells present atypical features which are similar to those of renal cell carcinoma (Fig. 5.6a–c).

Key features:

- Predominantly macrophages
- Epithelial cells from cyst lining
- Rarely, round lamellated structures (Liesegang rings)

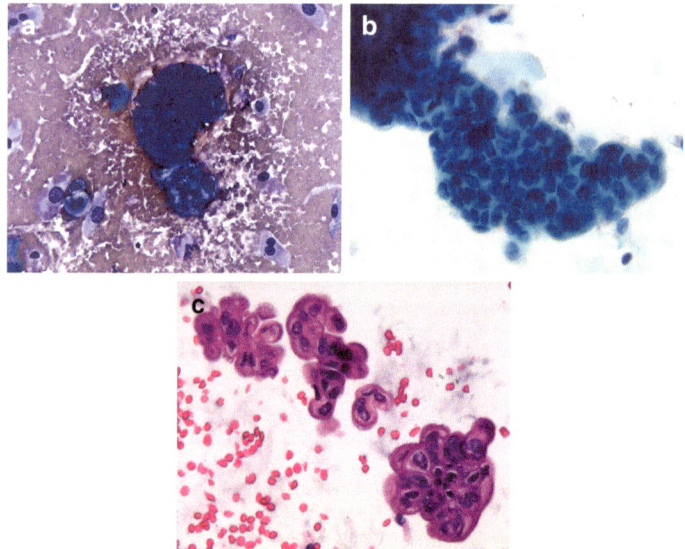

FIG. 5.6.   Benign cyst: Atypical epithelial fragments. In this case, a neoplasm was suspected, but the resected cyst was completely benign. (**a**) Epithelial tissue fragment (Diff-Quik stain, low power). (**b**) A large atypical epithelial fragment composed of disorganized epithelial cells with enlarged nuclei slightly varying in size and shape (Papanicolaou stain, medium power). (**c**) Atypical tissue fragments (H&E stain, medium power)

Differential diagnosis:
In most cases the diagnosis can be made with the characteristic features seen in FNA samples. In rare cases, atypical cells may mimic renal cell carcinoma or cystic renal cell neoplasms with extensive necrosis may be misdiagnosed as benign cyst in aspiration material.

Extramedullary Hematopoiesis (EMH)

EMH occurs in conditions of decreased hematopoiesis by bone marrow or increased destruction of peripheral red blood cells and commonly presents as diffuse involvement of liver and spleen. The occurrence of EMH as a solitary mass in the kidney is rare. Malignancy is usually suspected on imaging studies, and diagnosis is made by FNA or core biopsy.

In FNA specimens, the presence of erythroid and myelocytic precursor cells and megakaryocytes in correlation with clinical features, blood and bone marrow findings, establishes the diagnosis.

Benign Neoplasms

Oncocytoma

Oncocytomas comprise 3–5 % of primary renal tumors in adults. The majority occur over the age of 50 and predominantly in men. Approximately two-thirds are found incidentally by imaging studies performed for unrelated reasons. They are generally solitary lesions, but multiple, unilateral, or bilateral tumors occur in 5–6 % of cases.

Histologically, oncocytomas are usually composed of nests of oncocytic cells with eosinophilic, granular cytoplasm and typically round, uniform nuclei with evenly dispersed, finely granular chromatin (Fig. 5.7a). Occasional large, pleomorphic nuclei can be found in some cases.

Cytomorphology:
FNA samples usually reveal varying sizes of tissue fragments and cell aggregates as well as some single cells with oncocytic features (Fig. 5.7b). Typically tumor cells have uniform, round nuclei with or without prominent nucleoli (Fig. 5.7c). Occasional large, pleomorphic nuclei may be present in some cases. Cytoplasm is usually abundant, homogeneous, and finely granular.

Immunohistochemistry:
Oncocytomas are positive for AE1/AE3, CAM5.2, CD117, Ksp-cadherin, and negative for CAIX, CK7, Ep-CAM, and RCC.

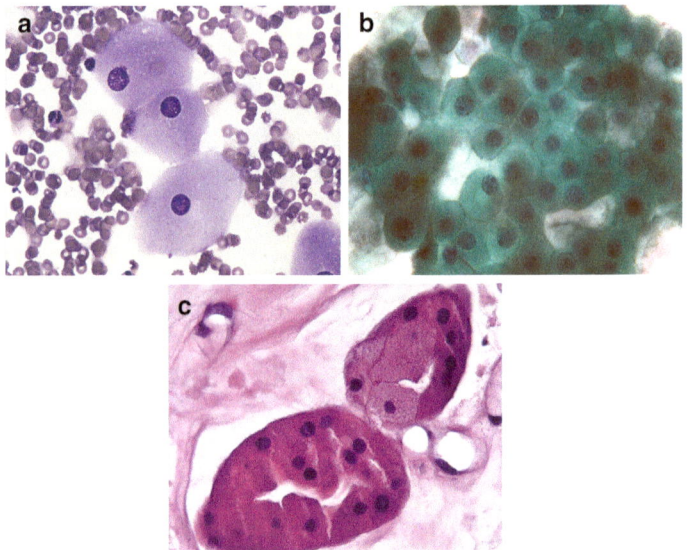

Fig. 5.7.   Oncocytoma: (**a**) Large cells with round, central, or eccentric nuclei with prominent nucleoli. (Diff-Quik stain, high power).
(**b**) Large oncocytic cells with round, uniform nuclei, prominent
nucleoli, and granular cytoplasm. (Papanicolaou stain, high power).
(**c**) Oncocytic cells forming two glandular structures. (Cell block,
H&E stain)

Key features:

- Uniform tumor cell population with homogeneous, acido-
philic, granular cytoplasm
- Uniform, round nuclei with smooth outlines with or without prominent nucleoli

Differential diagnosis:

Other types of RCC with areas of oncocytic differentiation
should be ruled out. Multiple biopsies (FNA and core) from
different areas of the tumor minimize sampling error. In limited material, cytopathologic diagnosis should be made
cautiously indicating that the findings are consistent with
oncocytoma if the findings are representative of the entire

tumor. Chromophobe (CR) RCC with predominantly eosinophilic cell component can be misdiagnosed as oncocytoma. CRRCC has nuclei with wrinkled borders, variation in size, and frequent binucleation.

Positive perinuclear staining with Hale's colloidal iron stain is typical for CRRCC and helps in its differentiation from oncocytoma.

Angiomyolipoma

Angiomyolipoma is a benign mesenchymal neoplasm composed of varying proportions of epithelioid smooth muscle cells, fat, and blood vessels with thick walls. It comprises about 2 % of renal neoplasms. Although the majority of renal angiomyolipomas are sporadic, there is a strong association with tuberous sclerosis. Between 75 and 80 % of patients with tuberous sclerosis develop angiomyolipomas. Angiomyolipomas can be accurately diagnosed by imaging studies, with the exception of a small proportion with absence of or a small amount of fat tissue which do not have the characteristic imaging features. Many morphological variants have been described. One variant, epithelioid angiomyolipoma, is considered potentially malignant. Local invasion and rare cases of metastases have been reported.

Cytomorphology:
Varying proportions of adipose tissue, spindle and epithelioid cells with rare intranuclear inclusions can be identified (Fig. 5.8a, b). Thick-walled blood vessels can only be seen in cell blocks and core biopsies (Fig. 5.8c).

Immunohistochemistry:
Muscle markers (SMA, desmin), vimentin, c-kit, and HMB45 are usually positive (Fig. 5.8d).

Key features:

- Mixture of adipose tissue, atypical epithelioid cells, and spindle cells
- Thick-walled blood vessels (cell block or core biopsy)
- Focal positive HMB45 staining

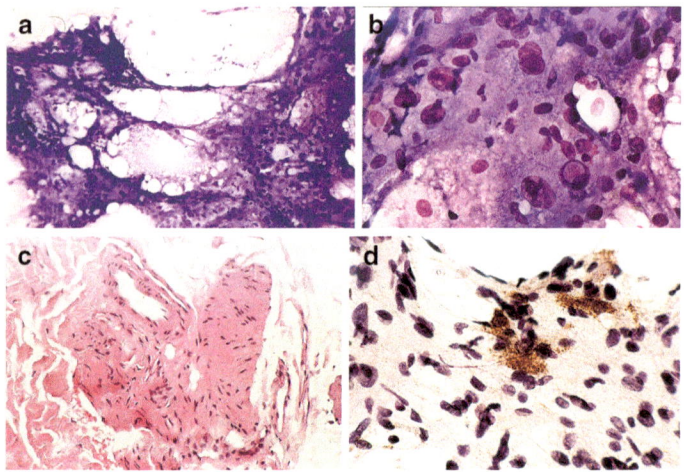

Fig. 5.8.   Angiomyolipoma: (**a**) Adipose tissue and epithelioid cells. (Diff-Quik stain, low power) (**b**) Atypical epithelial smooth muscle cells: large nuclei with prominent nucleoli, one intranuclear pseudoinclusion (Diff-Quik stain, medium power) (**c**) Thick walled blood vessels (Cell block, H&E stain, low power) (**d**) Positive staining with HMB45. (Medium power)

Differential diagnosis:
Cases of predominantly atypical epithelioid cells can be difficult to differentiate from high-grade, poorly differentiated primary or metastatic carcinomas. Immunostains could be helpful as could repeat FNA and/or core biopsies with extensive sampling of the tumor and correlation of clinical and radiological findings.

Metanephric Adenoma

A rare benign neoplasm of kidney, generally occurring in adults but also seen in children. Most of these tumors are discovered incidentally during investigations for other problems requiring abdominal imaging studies. Histologically the tumor is composed of small epithelial cells forming small acini and lobulated papillary formations.

Cytomorphology:
There are a few publications about FNA of this tumor reporting cellular specimens composed of oval to round cells are arranged in microfollicular and papillary pattern. The tumor cells have scant cytoplasm, uniform nuclei with evenly distributed fine chromatin and, occasionally, small nucleoli. No pleomorphism, necrosis, or mitosis is present.

Immunohistochemistry:
Tumor cells are reported to be positive for vimentin, WT1, and CD57.

Key features:

• Cellular specimen
• Small cells with scant cytoplasm forming small acini

Differential diagnosis:
Solid forms of papillary renal cell carcinoma, nephroblastoma, and metastatic carcinomas such as papillary carcinoma of thyroid are major tumors to be considered in the differential diagnosis. Immunostain TTF-1 is positive in thyroid carcinoma and negative in metanephric tumor.

Malignant Neoplasms

Kidney cancers usually occur in older people. They may be sporadic or hereditary. The latter comprise about 4 % of kidney tumors. The majority of these primary malignant neoplasms of kidney are carcinomas arising from renal parenchyma. Primary tumors arising from the renal pelvis are rare. They are mostly urothelial, but squamous cell and adenocarcinomas may also occur.

Renal Cell Carcinomas (RCCs)

Renal cell carcinomas make up a small percentage (~3 %) of adult malignancies. They have multiple chromosomal abnormalities which differ among the types of RCCs. Some of these

TABLE 5.1.   Genetic abnormalities in primary renal carcinomas.

Type of neoplasm	Genetic abnormality
Clear Cell (conventional) RCC	3p deletions
	Mutations of VHL gene
	Deletions of 6q, 8p, 9p, 14q
Papillary RCC	Trisomies of 3q, 7, 8, 12, 16, 17, 20
	Loss of Y
Chromophobe RCC	Monosomy of 1, 2, 6, 10, 13, 17, 21
	Hypodiploid DNA
Collecting duct carcinoma	Losses of 1, 6, 14, 15, 22
	Deletions of 8p and 13q
Mucinous tubular and spindle cell carcinoma	Loss of chromosomes 1, 4, 6, 8, 9, 13, 15, 22

TABLE 5.2.   Types of primary renal carcinomas.

Clear cell (conventional) RCC
Papillary RCC
Chromophobe RCC
Collecting duct carcinoma
Medullary RCC
Mucinous Tubular and Spindle Cell Carcinoma
Renal Cell Carcinoma with Xp11.2 Translocation
Unclassified RCC

are shown in Table 5.1 Three major types, conventional (clear cell), papillary, and chromophobe, comprise 85–90 % of RCCs. There is limited information about FNA findings in the remaining rare types, some of which will be covered in addition to the major types (Table 5.2).

Grading of RCC

Fuhrman grading is used in surgically resected specimens for predicting prognosis. The grades are based on nuclear size, nuclear shape, and size of nucleoli. Grade I, round uniform nuclei, approximately 10 μm, inconspicuous or absent nucleoli; Grade II, larger nuclei, approximately 15 μm, with irregular outlines, prominent nucleoli using ×40 objective; Grade III, larger nuclei, approximately 20 μm, with markedly

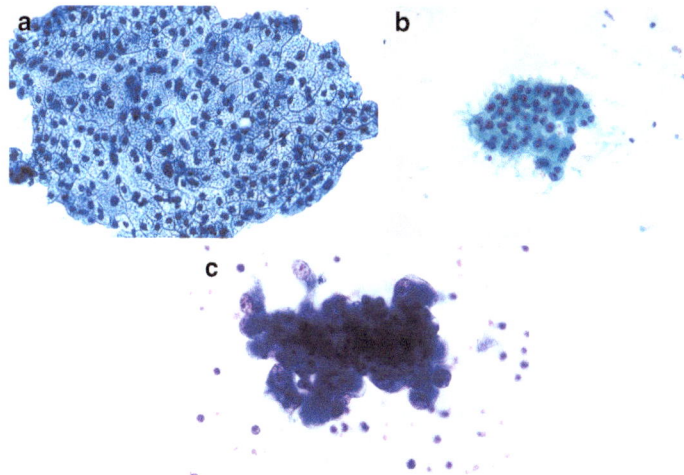

Fɪɢ. 5.9.   Clear cell (conventional) renal cell carcinoma (CCCRCC): Grading of RCC. (**a**) Low grade RCC (Fuhrman Gr. 1–2). Uniform, round nuclei with slight variation in size, inconspicuous nucleoli. (**b**) High grade RCC (Fuhrman Gr. 3). Large nuclei with macronucleoli. (**c**) High grade RCC (Fuhrman Gr. 4). Large pleomorphic nuclei with large nucleoli. (**a–c**, Papanicolaou stain, low power). (**a, c**) Reprinted with permission from: Fine Needle Aspiration Cytology, eds. MK Sidawy, SZ Ali, Churchill Livingston/Elsevier, 2007, Chapter 10, Kidney and Adrenal Glands, YS Erozan, pages 299–346

irregular borders and prominent nucleoli using ×10 objective; Grade IV, markedly atypical nuclei, larger than 20 μm, prominent nucleoli using ×10 objective, and often spindle cell component (Fig. 5.9a–c). Grade I and Grade IV tumors are rare in most series.

Agreement between the grading in needle biopsy specimens, both core biopsies and FNAs, and grading in surgical resected specimens has been found to be moderate, with biopsy specimens having a tendency to undergrading. The difference may be explained by the grading of surgical specimens being based on the area showing the highest grade of changes.

Accuracy of FNA in the Diagnosis of RCCs

FNAs are highly accurate for the diagnosis of RCCs. Subtypes of RCC are also diagnosed with very high accuracy in clear cell type. The accuracy of correct identification of papillary RCC and chromophobe RCC varies in published series.

Clear Cell (Conventional) Renal Cell Carcinoma (CRCC)

Clear cell (conventional) is the most common subtype, comprising 70 % of renal cell carcinomas. Sporadic CRCCs are usually solitary tumors. Multiple, bilateral tumors are rare in sporadic CRCC, but they are typical of hereditary forms such as Von Hippel–Lindau syndrome.

Histologically, the tumor is comprised of polygonal or cuboidal cells with clear or granular cytoplasm and distinct cytoplasmic borders surrounded by a thin-walled vascular network. Cytoplasm of clear cells contains lipid and glycogen. Various architectural patterns, including pseudopapillary forms, can be seen. Cystic changes, hemorrhage, and necrosis are common.

Cytomorphology:
Ultrasound- or CT-guided FNAs with on-site evaluation yield cellular material composed predominantly of tissue fragments and cell clusters (Fig. 5.10a, b). Tumor cells have clear or finely vacuolated cytoplasm with distinct cellular cytoplasmic borders (Fig. 5.11a, b). Most of the tumors have small round nuclei with inconspicuous or small nucleoli which correspond to Fuhrman Grade 2 (Fig. 5.11b). Higher grade tumors have larger nuclei with prominent nucleoli (Fig. 5.11c). One of the characteristic cytopathologic features of this tumor is crossing delicate vasculature in the tissue fragments (Fig. 5.12). Pseudopapillary fragments may be seen. They lack the fibrovascular stalk of the true papillary formations found in papillary renal cell carcinomas.

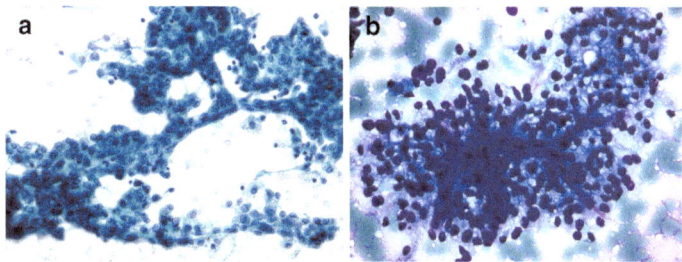

Fɪɢ. 5.10.   Clear cell (conventional) renal cell carcinoma: (**a**) A large tissue fragment with focal glandular formations. Tumor cells have enlarged nuclei, slightly varying in size with inconspicuous nucleoli and moderate to large amounts of dense cytoplasm. (Papanicolaou stain, low power) (**b**) Another large tissue fragment composed of tumor cells with large, vacuolated cytoplasm. (Diff-Quik, low power)

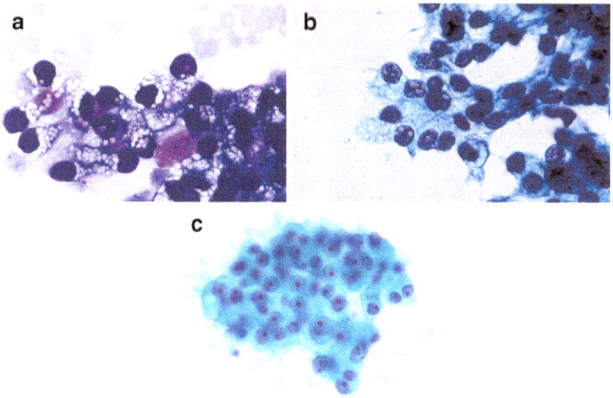

Fɪɢ. 5.11.   Clear cell (conventional) renal cell carcinoma: Vacuoles. (**a**) (Diff-Quik, high power). (**b**) Tumor cells have enlarged nuclei with irregular borders, coarse chromatin pattern, prominent nucleoli, and dense vacuolated cytoplasm. (Papanicolaou stain, high power). (**c**) Clear cell (conventional) renal cell carcinoma—High grade. Enlarged, round nuclei with bland chromatin and smooth nuclear borders. This tumor is high grade because of the macronucleoli. (Papanicolaou stain, high power). Reprinted with permission from: Fine Needle Aspiration Cytology, eds. MK Sidawy, SZ Ali, Churchill Livingston/Elsevier, 2007, Chapter 10, Kidney and Adrenal Glands, YS Erozan, pages 299–346

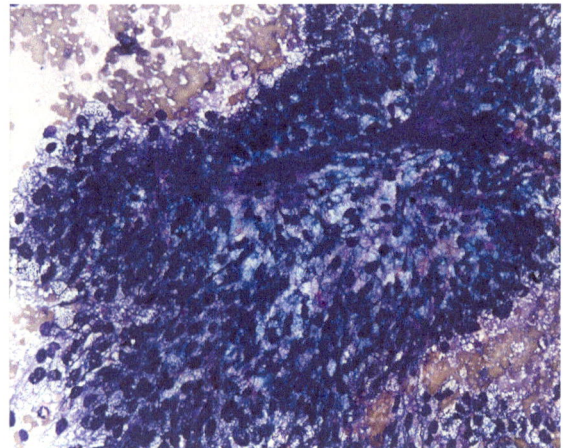

FIG. 5.12.   Clear cell (conventional) renal cell carcinoma: A large tissue fragment of tumor with crossing vessels. (Diff-Quik, low power)

Immunohistochemistry:
CRCC is usually positive for AE1/AE3 keratins, vimentin, RCC, CD10, CAIX, PAX-8, PAX-2 and negative for CD117, Ksp-cadherin, and parvalbumin.

Key features:

• Cellular specimen with predominantly tissue fragments
• Neoplastic cells with clear or finely vacuolated cytoplasm
• Tissue fragments of tumor with transgressing thin-walled blood vessels

Differential diagnosis:
The most important differential diagnosis is the differentiation of CRCC from metastatic tumors with clear cell features. Adrenal cortical carcinoma and hepatocellular carcinoma are among these neoplasms. Papillary carcinomas with focal clear cell changes should also be considered. In the absence of clear cell changes, oncocytoma and chromophobe RCC may enter into the differential diagnoses.

Papillary Renal Cell Carcinoma (PRCC)

Papillary renal cell carcinoma comprises 10–15 % of renal parenchymal neoplasms. They are three times more common in men than in women. More than half of these neoplasms are discovered incidentally by abdominal ultrasound or computed tomography performed for other purposes. Multiple tumors are more common than conventional type. The survival rate, generally, is better than for conventional RCCs. The application of Fuhrman grading for prognoses is controversial. Genetically they show trisomy of chromosomes 7 and 17, with loss of the Y chromosome.

Characteristic histological features are papillary structures lined with neoplastic cells. Solid papillary and tubulopapillary forms are common. Aggregates of foamy histiocytes in the fibrovascular cores and hemosiderin pigment in the tumor cells and histiocytes are typically found. Two types have been classified: Type 1, the most common, composed of a single layer of neoplastic cells with scant, eosinophilic cytoplasm, small ovoid nuclei, and inconspicuous nucleoli. Abundant psammoma bodies may be seen. Type 2 tumors are composed of tumor cells with abundant eosinophilic cytoplasm with higher grade nuclei.

Cytomorphology:
Diagnostic FNA specimens are hypercellular, comprised predominantly of tissue fragments, cellular aggregates, and some single cells. There are usually some tissue fragments with characteristic papillary formation (Fig. 5.13), fibrovascular core surrounded by neoplastic cells which exhibit scant to moderate amounts of cytoplasm and round or ovoid nuclei with inconspicuous or small nucleoli (Fig. 5.14). Varying proportions of neoplastic cells may have clear cell features. Globular forms and loose cellular aggregates can be the predominant component (Fig. 5.15). The presence of abundant psammoma bodies is one of the characteristic features of these neoplasms (Fig. 5.14). Foamy histiocytes and hemosiderin pigment in tumor cells and histiocytes (Fig. 5.16a–c) are characteristic features of papillary RCC which help to

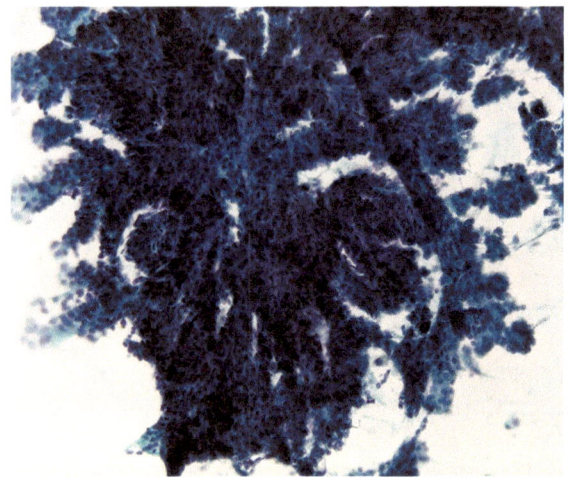

F<small>IG</small>. 5.13. Papillary carcinoma: Large papillary fragment. (Papanicolaou stain, low power)

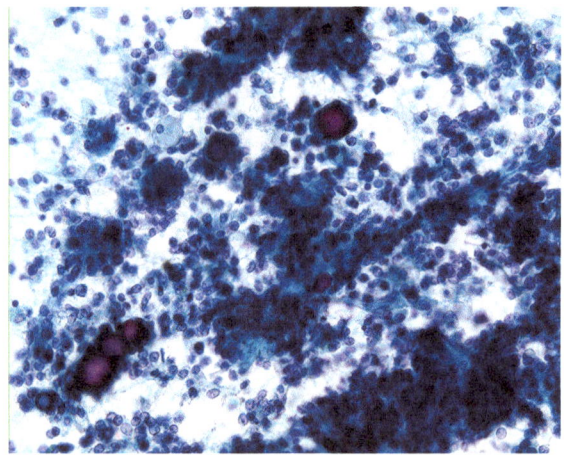

F<small>IG</small>. 5.14. Papillary renal cell carcinoma: Papillary structures, single cells, and multiple psammoma bodies. (Papanicolaou stain, medium power)

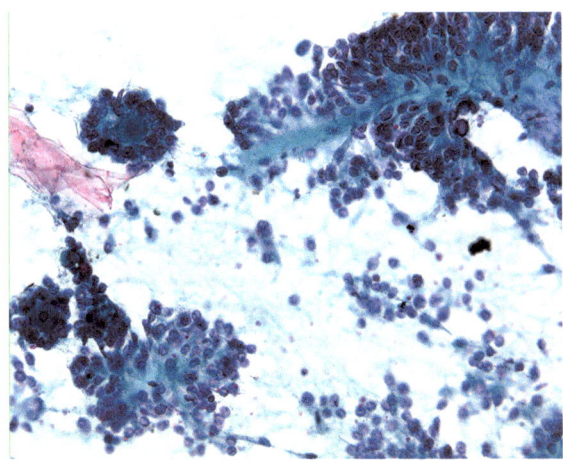

FIG. 5.15.   Papillary renal cell carcinoma: A papillary fragment with fibrovascular core and two globular structures forming psammoma bodies. (Papanicolaou stain, medium power)

differentiate this tumor from other types of RCCs. Clear cell features, focally or predominantly, could be present.

Immunohistochemistry (IHC):
IHC is performed on the cell blocks or core biopsies. Papillary RCCs are strongly and diffusely positive for CK7 and AMACR (cytoplasmic, granular) and also positive for RCC, PAX-2, PAX-8, and CD10 (Fig. 5.17a–c).

Key features:

- Hypercellular specimen with predominantly tissue fragments
- Papillary forms with fibrovascular stalk
- Neoplastic cells having round or ovoid nuclei with inconspicuous nucleoli and scant to moderate cytoplasm (Type 1)
- Histiocytes, single or in aggregates
- Hemosiderin pigment in histiocytes and neoplastic cells
- Psammoma bodies, often abundant
- Less frequently, large nuclei with prominent nucleoli and moderate to large amounts of cytoplasm (Type 2)

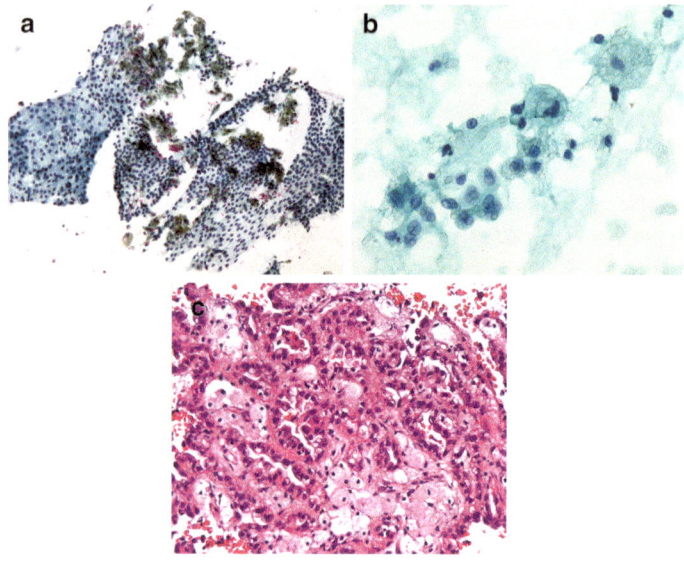

FIG. 5.16.   Papillary renal cell carcinoma: (**a**) Monolayer fragments
of papillary carcinoma with hemosiderin pigment in the tumor cells
and histiocytes. (Papanicolaou stain, low power) (**b**) A group of
tumor cells and histiocytes. A few tumor cells have *green* intracytoplasmic hemosiderin pigment. (Papanicolaou stain, high power) (**c**)
Tightly packed histiocytes surrounded by tumor cell. (Cell block,
H&E stain, medium power)

Differential diagnosis:

The characteristic cytomorphology includes papillary structures with foamy hemosiderin-laden histiocytes and hemosiderin pigment in the tumor cells. When the papillary tumor is
composed of predominantly clear cells, the differential diagnosis includes mainly clear cell RCC and other rare subtypes,
clear cell papillary RCC, and Xp11.2 translocation RCC. The
presence of hemosiderin pigment in tumor cells, hemosiderin-laden histiocytes, and psammoma bodies are helpful
features in differentiating PRCC from other renal neoplasms
with clear cell features. Immunohistochemical and genetic
profiles of these neoplasms are also different from PRCC.

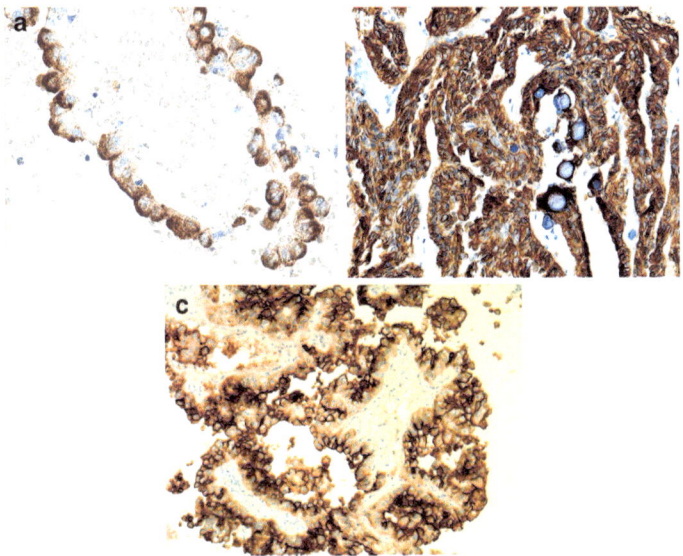

FIG. 5.17.   Papillary renal cell carcinoma: Cell block. Immunostains: (**a**) Strong reaction to RCC antibody. (H&E stain, low power) (**b**) Diffuse cytoplasmic staining with CK7 antibody. (low power) (**c**) Dense peripheral cytoplasmic staining with CD10 antibody. (low power). (**a**) Reprinted with permission from: Fine Needle Aspiration Cytology, eds. MK Sidawy, SZ Ali, Churchill Livingston/Elsevier, 2007, Chapter 10, Kidney and Adrenal Glands, YS Erozan, pages 299–346

Chromophobe Renal Cell Carcinoma

Chromophobe renal cell carcinoma (CRRCC) is a rare tumor comprising only about 5 % of renal cell carcinomas. Histologically, the tumor has two cell types: one has abundant clear to pale cytoplasm and the other granular, eosinophilic cytoplasm with thick cytoplasmic borders (eosinophilic type). Nuclei with wrinkled borders (raisinoid nuclei) and perinuclear clearing are characteristic features. Binucleation is common (Fig. 5.18).

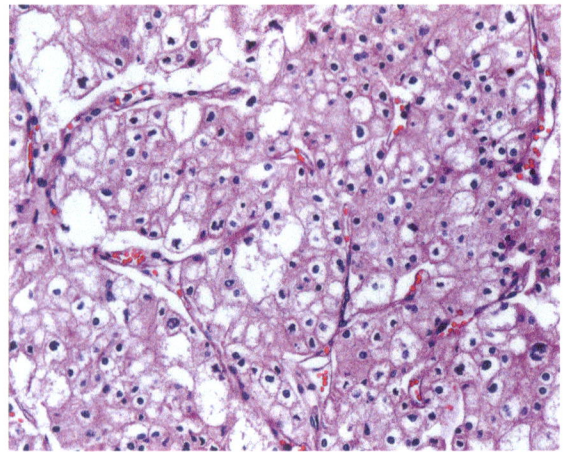

FIG. 5.18.   Chromophobe renal cell carcinoma: Tumor cells with eosinophilic, granular, pale or clear cytoplasm and hyperchromatic nuclei with irregular borders. Nuclei vary in size and most have clear areas surrounding the nucleus. Resected tumor. (H&E stain, medium power)

Cytomorphology:
FNA specimens are cellular with cohesive aggregates and single tumor cells (Fig. 5.19a). The latter have large pale or dense granular cytoplasm (Fig. 5.19b). Frequent binucleation and variation in nuclear size are characteristic features. Irregular nuclear borders and occasional intranuclear pseudoinclusions are also seen (Fig. 5.19c). The perinuclear clearing seen in histologic preparations is less apparent in cytologic preparations (Fig. 5.18).

Immunohistochemistry:
Chromophobe cell RCCs express AE1/AE3, CK7, EMA, parvalbumin, and Ksp-cadherin. Vimentin, CAIX, and AMACR are negative.

Key features:

• Small and large cells with clear, pale granular cytoplasm with thick cellular membrane

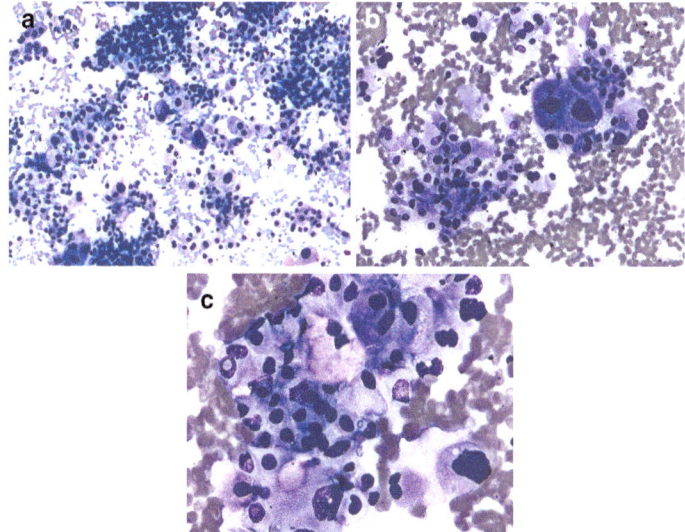

F<small>IG</small>. 5.19.   Chromophobe renal cell carcinoma: (**a**) Tissue fragments and single tumor cells. Marked variation in nuclear and cell size. Irregular nuclear borders and perinuclear clearing seen in some of the cells. (Diff-Quik stain, low power) (**b**) Binucleation, anisonucleosis, irregular nuclear borders, and a thin rim of perinuclear clearing in some cells. (Diff-Quik stain, high power) (**c**) Intranuclear pseudoinclusion. Marked anisonucleosis. (Diff-Quik stain, high power). (**c**) Reprinted with permission from: Fine Needle Aspiration Cytology, eds. MK Sidawy, SZ Ali, Churchill Livingston/Elsevier, 2007, Chapter 10, Kidney and Adrenal Glands, YS Erozan, pages 299–346

- Anisonucleosis and binucleation
- Irregular nuclear borders (raisinoid nuclei)

Differential diagnosis:
Oncocytoma and clear cell RCC have some overlapping cytomorphological features with CRRCC. Variation in nuclear size and irregularities in nuclear borders are helpful features in distinguishing these tumors from oncocytomas. Hale's colloidal iron stain is positive in CRRCC (perinuclear staining) but negative in oncocytoma and CRCC.

Collecting Duct Carcinoma (CDC)

Collecting duct carcinoma is a rare neoplasm comprising about 1 % of these tumors. The majority of the patients are in the fourth to seventh decade of life. Men are twice as commonly affected as women. CDC is a very aggressive tumor which is usually diagnosed in its advanced stage.

Cytomorphology:
There are only a few publications in the literature describing the cytopathologic findings in this tumor. In fine needle aspirates, the tumor is composed of tissue fragments, solid and pseudopapillary forms, and single cells. Fragments of dense fibrous tissue may also be present. Tumor cells have large nuclei with coarse granular chromatin, irregular borders, and prominent nucleoli. The cytoplasm is finely vacuolated in most tumor cells, but single large vacuoles are also seen in some (Fig. 5.20a, b). Intracytoplasmic mucin can be present. In the pleural and ascitic fluids, papillary structures with psammoma bodies have been reported.

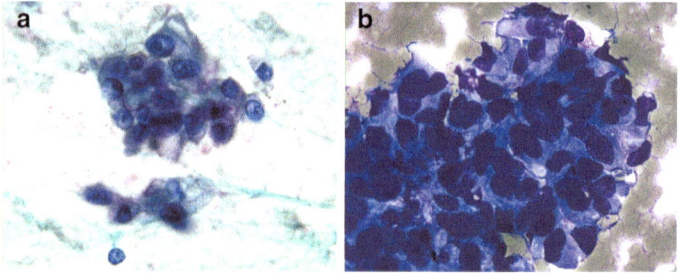

Fig. 5.20.   Collecting duct carcinoma: Poorly differentiated carcinoma with rare intracytoplasmic vacuoles. (**a**) (Papanicolaou stain, medium power). (**b**) (Diff-Quik stain, high power). (**a**) Reprinted with permission from: Fine Needle Aspiration Cytology, eds. MK Sidawy, SZ Ali, Churchill Livingston/Elsevier, 2007, Chapter 10, Kidney and Adrenal Glands, YS Erozan, pages 299–346

Immunohistochemistry:
Histologically the tumor is composed of neoplastic cells with pleomorphic nuclei forming irregular tubular or tubulopapillary structures associated with a fibrous stroma and inflammatory cell infiltrate.

Immunohistochemically, the tumor expresses characteristics of the collecting duct of the distal nephron. CDC shows a positive reaction to Ulex europaeus agglutinin-(UEA-1), peanut lectin, e-cadherin, pancytokeratins, high molecular cytokeratins, vimentin, and EMA. Reaction to markers for proximal tubules, such as CD10, RCC, and AMACR, is negative.

Key features:

- Aggressive tumor with poor prognosis
- Tissue fragments and single cells in FNA specimens
- Large nuclei with irregular borders and prominent nucleoli

Differential diagnosis:
Differential diagnosis includes other high-grade renal cell carcinomas and metastatic, poorly differentiated malignant neoplasms. Positive immunostaining with HMWCK and UEA-1 is helpful in differentiating this tumor from other renal cell neoplasms.

Medullary Renal Cell Carcinoma (MRCC)

Medullary renal cell carcinoma is a rare, highly aggressive neoplasm occurring in young, predominantly African-American, individuals with sickle cell trait. It is usually discovered in its advanced stage. Histologically, the tumor is described as having a yolk sac-like pattern, but solid nests or tubules can be seen. A polymorphonuclear leukocytic infiltrate is commonly present. Tumor cells have large, pleomorphic nuclei with macronucleoli and moderate to large amounts of eosinophilic cytoplasm.

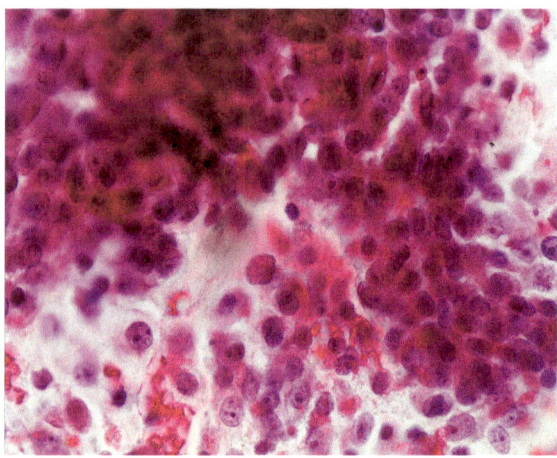

Fig. 5.21.   Medullary carcinoma: Tumor cells with large nuclei and prominent nucleoli. (H&E stain, medium power) (Courtesy of Srinivas R. Mandavilli, M.D.)

Cytomorphology:
There are a few case reports describing the cellular features of this tumor in FNAs and renal pelvic washings. In FNA specimens, the tumor cells occur as tissue fragments of loosely cohesive aggregates and single cells. Tumor cells have large nuclei with irregular borders and prominent nucleoli (Fig. 5.21). Single cells have eccentrically placed nuclei with eosinophilic cytoplasm and occasional intracytoplasmic vacuoles. Single cells with rhabdoid features are also present in some cases.

Special stains and immunohistochemistry:
Intracytoplasmic mucin is present in about three quarters of the tumors. Immunohistochemical stains show positive reactions to *U. europaeus* lectin, high molecular weight cytokeratin, and CK7. Tumor cells are nonreactive to Ksp-cadherin.

Key features:

- Tissue fragments, loosely cohesive cell aggregates, and single cells
- Neoplastic cells with high n/c ratio, large nuclei, and prominent nucleoli
- Intracytoplasmic mucin vacuoles
- Neoplastic cells with rhabdoid features in some cases

Differential diagnosis:
High-grade primary carcinomas of kidney, specifically collecting duct carcinomas and metastatic poorly differentiated carcinomas, should be considered in the differential diagnosis. Collecting duct carcinoma has many overlapping morphologic and immunohistochemical features with medullary carcinoma, making the differential diagnosis between these two entities impossible in needle biopsy specimens. The patient's clinical profile and immunostains help with the differential diagnosis.

Mucinous Tubular and Spindle Cell Carcinoma

Renal mucinous tubular and spindle cell carcinoma (RMTSCC) is a rare, low-grade renal neoplasm. Histologically, the tumor shows interconnecting tubular forms and spindle cells in myxoid stroma. Tumor cells have uniform, low-grade nuclei and vacuolated cytoplasm.

Cytomorphology:
Limited information is available in the literature on the cytopathologic characteristics of RMTSCC. Based on two case reports, FNA samples are described as cellular and composed of thick tissue fragments or loosely cohesive clusters and single cells. Tumor cells have round or oval, relatively uniform nuclei. Prominent nucleoli may be present. The cytoplasm is delicate and finely vacuolated.

Immunohistochemistry:
Positive for vimentin, CK7, AMACR, and EMA; negative for HMWCK, PAX-2, CD10, and RCC.

Cytogenetics:
Loss of chromosomes 1, 4, 6, 8, 9, 13, 15, and 22.

Key features:

- Cellular specimens composed of thick tissue fragments or cellular groups
- Tumor cells having round or ovoid nuclei with prominent nucleoli
- Delicate finely vacuolated cytoplasm

Differential diagnosis:
Clear cell and papillary renal cell carcinomas are the major types of RCCs in the differential diagnosis.

Renal Cell Carcinoma with Xp11.2 Translocation

The renal cell carcinomas in this entity are characterized by gene fusion of transcription factor E3 (TFE3), which is located on chromosome Xp11.2, with one of a number of variant partner genes.

These tumors commonly occur in pediatric and adolescent age groups, comprising one-third of the pediatric renal tumors. In adults, it is reported at 1.6 and 4.2 % of renal neoplasms in two series. Histologically, the tumor exhibits clear cell and papillary architecture or is a granular eosinophilic neoplasm with solid, nested, focally acinar, or tubular forms. Tumors with papillary architecture may have numerous psammoma bodies. Tumors with the ASPL-TFE3 gene fusion are associated with large cells having abundant cytoplasm, nuclei with vesicular chromatin, and prominent nucleoli arranged in alveolar or pseudopapillary forms. Many psammoma bodies are also present. The tumors with the PRCC-TFE3 gene fusion, on the other hand, have tumor cells with less cytoplasm and a more nested pattern. Psammoma bodies in these tumors are few or absent.

Cytomorphology:

Very limited information is available in the literature concerning the cytopathologic findings. In a case report of FNA of a metastasis to lung, predominantly follicular and/ or pseudoacinar structures were found in both Diff-Quik and Papanicolaou stained slides. In Diff-Quik stain, a meta-chromatic, hyalinized central core was present in the center of follicular structures surrounded by fairly monomorphic cells having round to oval nuclei and high nuclear to cyto-plasm ratio. Some of the cells had clear cytoplasm. In Papanicolaou-stained slides, a second population of cells forming sheets and papillary structures were present. The tumor cells had nuclei with fine chromatin and discrete nucleoli. The cytoplasm was mostly granular, but some clear cells were present.

Immunohistochemistry:

Tumor cells are strongly reactive to vimentin and TFE3. They are consistently reactive to RCC marker and CD10. Reaction to cytokeratins and EMA varies.

Cytogenetics:

The two most common translocations are t(X;17)(p11.2;q25) and t(X;1)(p11.2;q21) with TFE3 fusion with genes ASPL and PRCC.

Key features:

- A rare type of renal neoplasm characterized by fusion of TFE3 with one of the variant partner genes.
- Cellular specimens with tissue fragments, loosely cohesive clusters, and single cells.
- Round or oval nuclei and delicate finely vacuolated cytoplasm.
- Immunoreactivity to TFE3.

Differential diagnosis:

The main differential diagnosis is with conventional RCC. The immunocytochemical profile, specifically reactivity to TFE3, is helpful in differentiating this tumor from RCC.

Unclassified RCC

This category includes the renal carcinomas which do not fit into one of the other RCC categories. In practice, tumors which have the histopathologic/cytopathologic features of two different types of tumors (e.g., oncocytoma and chromophobe RCC) and tumors for which a definitive diagnosis cannot be made are also put into this category.

Sarcomatoid RCC

Sarcomatoid RCC is not considered a separate type, but a sarcomatous transformation (spindle or pleomorphic forms) occurring in any of the subtypes of renal cell carcinoma. In large series, transformation rate is reported as 5–9 % in major types of RCC. The presence of sarcomatoid changes adversely affects the outcome.

Cytomorphology:
In addition to the original tumor cell type, the presence of spindle cells with atypical nuclei is present. The latter may be present as single cells, loose groups, or in a tissue fragment admixed with high grade epithelial component of the tumor (Fig. 5.22a–c). If there is no evidence of original RCC, the tumor should be diagnosed as "RCC-unclassified."

Immunohistochemistry:
Positive reaction to AE1/AE3 and EMA has been reported.

Key features:

- Atypical spindle cells and pleomorphic tumor cells
- Cells with features of the original tumor

Differential diagnosis:
Poorly differentiated primary or metastatic carcinomas and sarcomas should be considered in the differential diagnosis. Immunostains are usually needed for diagnosis. RCC, PAX-2, and PAX-8 are helpful in determining renal origin.

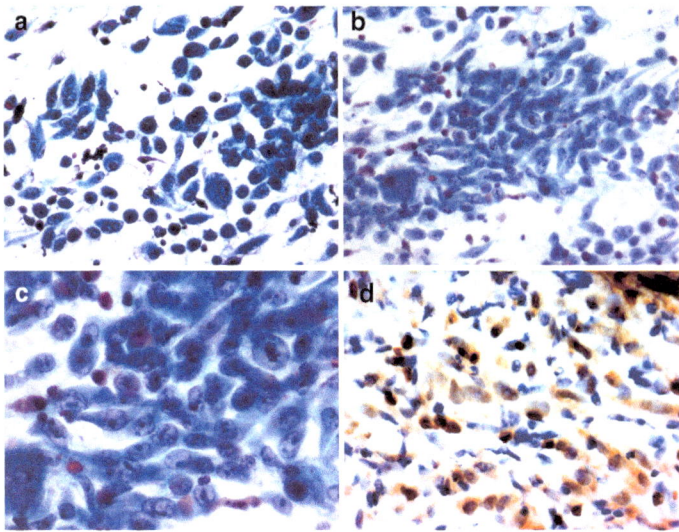

Fɪɢ. 5.22.   Sarcomatoid renal cell carcinoma: (**a**) Pleomorphic tumor cells, round, ovoid and spindle shapes, large nuclei with prominent nucleoli. Tumor cells vary from round cells with high nuclear to cytoplasmic ratio to large cells with unipolar extensions of cytoplasm. (Papanicolaou stain, medium power) (**b**) Predominantly spindle-shaped tumor cells with large nuclei and macronucleoli. (Papanicolaou stain, medium power) (**c**) Same as (**b**). Large nuclei with bland chromatin and macronucleoli. (Papanicolaou stain, high power (**d**) Cell block. Positive nuclear staining with antibody to PAX8. (High power)

Metastatic Neoplasms

Secondary neoplasms of kidney, although not uncommon in autopsy studies, are rare in FNAs of kidney. Most common tumors are carcinomas, specifically of lung, followed by lymphomas. In correlation with primary tumor diagnosis and adequate FNA samples, specific diagnosis can be made in almost all cases. On-site evaluation improves the adequacy of the specimen and helps to determine proper preparation techniques for the specific diagnosis.

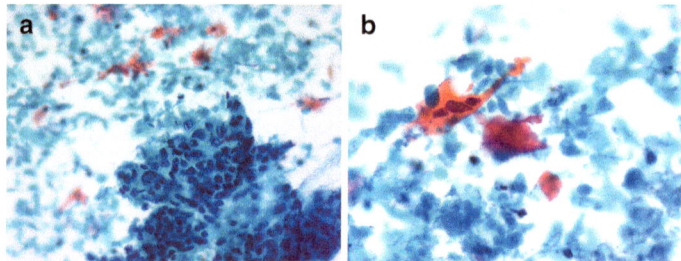

FIG. 5.23.   Metastatic squamous cell carcinoma, primary lung: (**a**) single keratinized cells and a nonkeratinized tissue fragment or squamous cell carcinoma in a necrotic background (Papanicolaou stain low power), (**b**) A multinucleated keratinized cancer cell. Nuclei vary in size and have irregular borders. (Papanicolaou stain, high power)

Cytomorphology:
FNA samples are usually cellular, and the morphology of the tumor is usually similar to the primary neoplasm. In poorly differentiated tumors, immunohistochemical stains may be required for the differential diagnosis between high-grade renal cell and urothelial carcinomas. Flow cytometry or immunohistochemistry is routinely used in lymphoma cases. Examples of metastatic carcinoma are shown in Figs. 5.23a, b, 5.24a, b, and 5.25a–c, and lymphoma in Fig. 5.26.

Urothelial Carcinoma of Renal Pelvis

Urothelial carcinoma is the most common type of malignant neoplasm (85–90 %) arising from the renal pelvis. Like urothelial carcinomas of bladder, they present as flat or papillary forms. They tend to be multifocal, occurring in other sites in the urinary tract.

Cytomorphology:
Cytologic samples are obtained by catheterization, renal pelvic washings, or, for large renal masses, FNA under US or CT

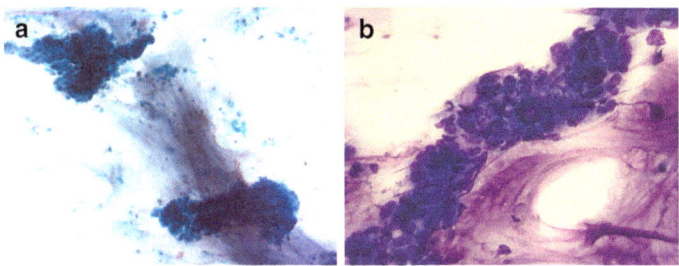

FIG. 5.24.   Metastatic adenocarcinoma, small intestine primary. (**a**) Two tissue fragments of tumor in mucinous background. (Papanicolaou stain, low power). (**b**) Two tissue fragments in mucinous background. The *lower fragment* is better differentiated having acinar formations. The one *above* is poorly differentiated, but has a single vacuole suggestive of adenocarcinoma. (Diff-Quik stain, high power)

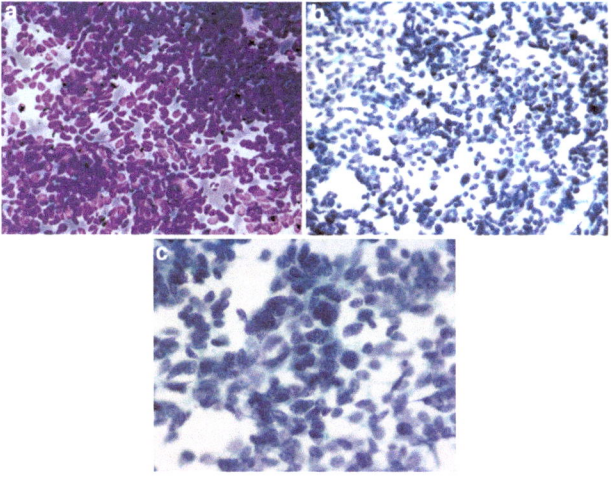

FIG. 5.25.   Small cell carcinoma: (**a** and **b**) Tumor cells have round or ovoid nuclei, some of which have sharp pointed ends. Cytoplasm is not visible in most. Frequent single cell "columns" or tumor cells with nuclear molding are present. (**a**) (Diff-Quik stain, medium power), (**b**) (Papanicolaou stain, medium power). (**c**) In addition to the features described above, an evenly dispersed fine granular chromatin pattern, characteristic of neuroendocrine neoplasms, is seen in many nuclei. (Papanicolaou stain, high power)

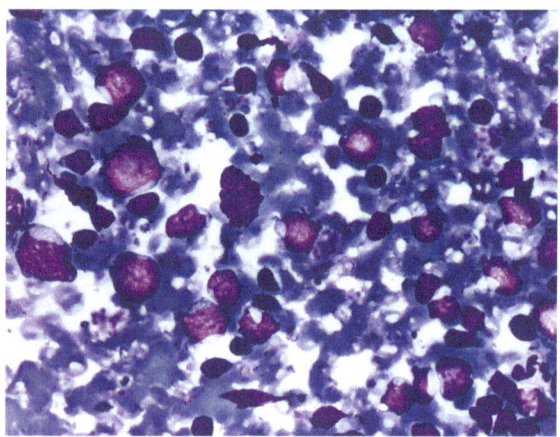

FIG. 5.26.   Large B cell lymphoma: Large, single cells with round nuclei and scanty cytoplasm. One cell has an eccentrically placed nucleus and irregular border. (Diff-Quik, high power)

guidance. The cytopathologic diagnosis of low grade urothelial carcinoma can be difficult, particularly in renal pelvic washings. High grade urothelial carcinomas are diagnosed with higher accuracy in both FNA and renal pelvic washings. Low-grade tumors appear as papillary tissue fragments and some single cells. High-grade urothelial carcinomas typically have an increased number of single tumor cells in addition to tissue fragments. Tumor cells have large, hyperchromatic nuclei and high nuclear to cytoplasmic (n:c) ratios (Figs. 5.27 and 5.28a–c). Focal glandular and squamous differentiation can be present.

Immunohistochemistry:
Immunostains for p63, p16(INK4a), GATA3, thrombomodulin, uroplakin, and HMWCK are positive.

Key features:

- Low grade urothelial carcinoma

    – Predominantly tissue fragments
    – Papillary forms
    – Uniform, round nuclei

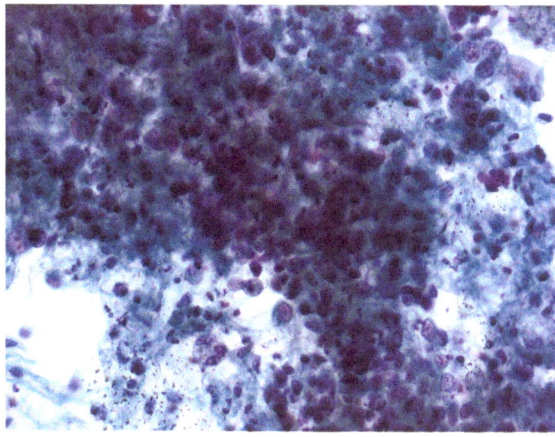

FIG. 5.27.   High grade urothelial carcinoma: Renal pelvic wash. A large tissue fragment and single tumor cell in a necrotic background. Tumor cells have large nuclei with prominent nucleoli and high nuclear to cytoplasmic ratio. (Papanicolaou stain, medium power)

- High grade urothelial carcinoma
    - Tissue fragments and single cells
    - Hyperchromatic nuclei with irregular borders
    - High n:c ratio
    - Mitoses

Differential diagnosis:
Poorly differentiated RCCs, collecting duct carcinoma, and poorly differentiated metastatic carcinomas should be considered among the differential diagnoses. Immunostains are helpful in differentiating urothelial carcinomas from other neoplasms.

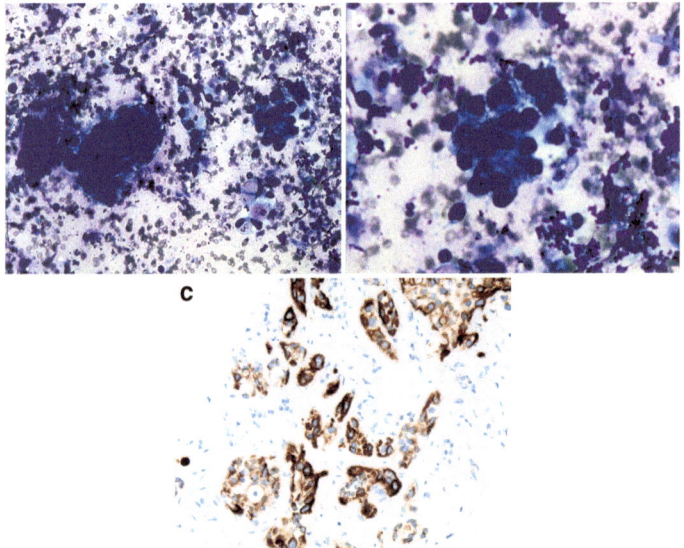

F<small>IG</small>. 5.28.   High grade urothelial carcinoma: FNA. (**a**) Several tissue
fragments and single cells. Although they are consistent with a carcinoma, the origin of the tumor cannot be established with certainty.
Presence of several tumor cells with large vacuoles and architecture
suggestive of glandular differentiation can be seen in both urothelial
and renal cell carcinomas. (Diff-Quik stain, medium power). (**b**)
Tissue fragment of tumor with features suggestive of glandular differentiation. (Diff-Quik stain, high power). (**c**) Core biopsy. Nests of
tumor. Positive immunostain CK903 supports the diagnosis of urothelial carcinoma versus renal cell carcinoma. (Low power)

Nephroblastoma (Wilms Tumor)

Nephroblastomas comprise about 80 % of pediatric malignant
renal neoplasms, and 98 % of them occur before age 10.
Histologically, nephroblastomas exhibit a triphasic pattern
composed of blastemal, epithelial, and stromal cell types in
varying proportions. However, monophasic and biphasic forms
frequently occur. Blastemal cells are small with scant cytoplasm. Tumor cells are closely packed with overlapping nuclei.

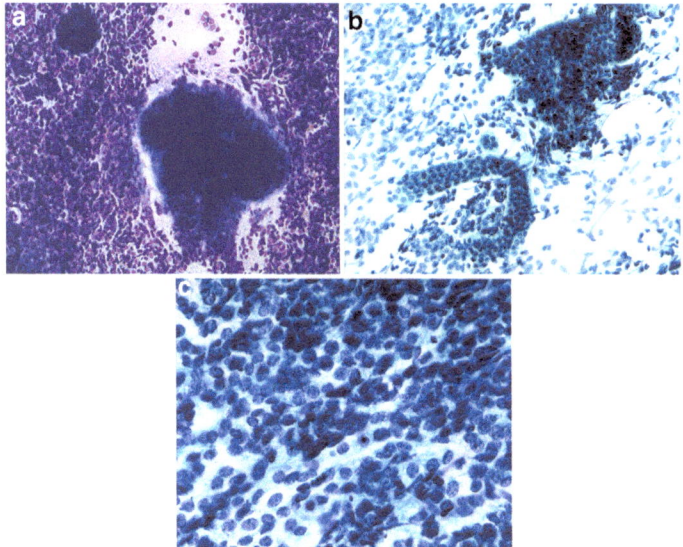

Fig. 5.29. Nephroblastoma (Wilms tumor): (**a**) Epithelial tissue fragments in a background of blastemal cells. (Diff-Quik, low power), (**b**) Epithelial, blastemal, and stromal (Spindle cells) components of tumor. (Papanicolaou stain, medium power). (**c**) Blastemal cells, round or ovoid nuclei, scant cytoplasm. (Papanicolaou stain, high power)

They form distinct patterns, most frequently nodular and serpentine. An epithelial component appears in tubular or papillary and, rarely, primitive rosette-like formations. A stromal component is usually composed of myxoid and spindle cells. Smooth and striated muscle and other types of stromal tissue, such as cartilage, osteoid, neuroglial, and adipose tissue, may be seen. Anaplastic nephroblastoma is a rare form of nephroblastoma characterized by marked nuclear atypia and multipolar polyploid mitotic figures.

Cytomorphology:
FNA specimens are usually cellular, containing predominantly blastemal cells with epithelial and stromal elements. In biphasic tumors, blastemal and epithelial cells are present (Fig. 5.29a, b). Epithelial elements are present in the form of

tubules, cords, rosettes, and sheets (Fig. 5.29b). Blastemal components are typically small cells with round nuclei and scant cytoplasm. The nuclei have fine granular, evenly dispersed chromatin. Nucleoli are absent (Fig. 5.29c). Immature glomerular formations may be present. Stromal elements can be scant and composed of spindle cells mixed with blastemal and epithelial elements.

Immunohistochemistry:
Blastemal cells are reactive to vimentin and desmin, but not primitive muscle markers such as MyoD1 and myogenin. Reaction for WT1 confined to nucleus is diffusely expressed in blastemal cells and early epithelial differentiation.

Key features:

- Presence of blastemal, epithelial, and stromal elements are diagnostic features
- Biphasic types, composed of blastemal and epithelial components, are common
- Monophasic types containing only one component may occur

Differential diagnosis:
Differential diagnoses for nephroblastoma are other pediatric renal neoplasms, mainly small round blue cell tumors which include neuroblastoma, congenital neuroblastic nephroma, primitive neuroectodermal tumor, and lymphoma.

Rhabdoid Tumor

This is a high-grade malignant neoplasm comprising 2.5 % of pediatric renal malignancies. More than 95 % of these tumors occur before the age of 3.

Cytomorphology:
FNA specimens are markedly cellular and contain varying proportions of rhabdoid cells occurring singly or in clusters. Characteristic features of rhabdoid cells are peripherally

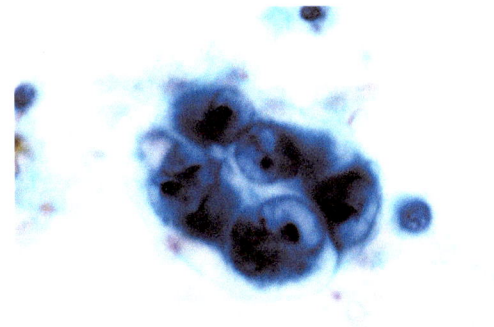

Fig. 5.30.   Rhabdoid tumor: A group of tumor cells with large eccentrically placed nuclei and macronucleoli. (Papanicolaou stain, high power) (Courtesy of Paul E. Wakely, Jr., M.D.)

placed, large nuclei with macronucleoli and moderate amounts of cytoplasm containing perinuclear global densities (Fig. 5.30). The latter correspond to areas of condensed microfilaments seen on electron microscopic examination. In addition to rhabdoid cells, atypical round cells with hyperchromatic nuclei, inconspicuous nucleoli, and scant to moderate cytoplasm are found in most cases. In rare cases, spindle-shaped tumor cells have also been described.

Immunohistochemistry and special stains:
Vimentin (+), CKs (+), INI1 (−), EMA (+), PAS (+) (Perinuclear densities.)

Key features:

• Rhabdoid cells with eccentric nuclei, macronucleoli, and cytoplasmic perinuclear global densities.
• Various proportions of round atypical cells, epithelial cells and, rarely, spindle-shaped tumor cells may be present.
• In the absence of characteristic rhabdoid cells, immunohistochemical and genetic studies may be needed to establish a diagnosis

Differential diagnosis:
Commonly, nephroblastoma with rhabdoid features. Rare variants of RCC are congenital mesoblastic nephroma, urothelial carcinoma, rhabdomyosarcoma, colleting duct carcinoma, oncocytoma, neuroepithelial tumor, and lymphoma.

Suggested Reading

General

Adeniran AJ, Al-Ahmadie H, Iyengar P, et al. Fine needle aspiration of renal cortical lesions in adults. Diagn Cytopathol. 2010;38: 710–5.

Andonian S, Okeke Z, VanderBrink BA, et al. Aetiology of non-diagnostic renal fine-needle aspiration cytologies in a contemporary series. BJU Int. 2009;103:28–32.

Brierly RD, Thomas PJ, Harrison NW, et al. Evaluation of fine-needle aspiration cytology for renal masses. BJU Int. 2000;85:14–8.

DeWitt J, Gress FG, Levy MJ, et al. EUS-guided FNA aspiration of kidney masses: a multicenter U.S. experience. Gastrointest Endosc. 2009;70:573–8.

Geisinger KR, Stanley MW, Raab SS, et al. Kidney. In: Modern cytopathology. New York: Churchill Livingstone Elsevier; 2004. p. 529–618.

Katz RL, Krishnamurthy S. Kidney, adrenal, and retroperitoneum. In: Bibbo M, Wilbur DC, editors. Comprehensive cytopathology. 3rd ed. Philadelphia: Saunders Elsevier; 2008. p. 811–71.

Murphy MW, Grignon DJ, Perlman EJ. Tumors of the kidney, bladder and related urinary structures. Atlas of tumor pathology, 4th series, Fascicle 1. Washington, DC: Armed Forces Institute of Pathology; 2004.

Srigley JR, Delahunt B, Eble JN, et al. The International Society of Urological Pathology (ISUP) Vancouver classification of renal neoplasia. Am J Surg Pathol. 2013;37:1469–89.

Truong ID, Todd TD, Dhurandhar B, et al. Fine-needle aspiration of renal masses in adults: analysis of results and diagnostic problems in 18 cases. Diagn Cytopathol. 1999;20:333–49.

Volpe A, Jewett MA. Current role, techniques and outcomes of percutaneous biopsy of renal tumors. Expert Rev Anticancer Ther. 2009;9:773–83.

Adequacy and Accuracy

Bishop JA, Hosler GA, Kulesza P, et al. Fine-needle aspiration of renal cell carcinoma: is accurate Fuhrman grading possible on cytologic material? Diagn Cytopathol. 2010;39:168–71.

Blumenfeld AJ, Guru K, Fuchs GJ, et al. Percutaneous biopsy of renal cell carcinoma underestimates nuclear grade. Urology. 2010;76:610–3.

Kummerlin IP, Smedts F, ten Kate FJ, et al. Cytological punctures in the diagnosis of renal tumours: a study on accuracy and reproducibility. Eur Urol. 2009;55:187–95.

Renshaw AA, Lee KR, Madge R, et al. Accuracy of fine needle aspiration in distinguishing subtypes of renal cell carcinoma. Acta Cytol. 1997;41:987–94.

Benign Lesions

Aydin H, Magi-Galluzzi C, Lane BR, et al. Renal angiomyolipoma: clinicopathologic study of 194 cases with emphasis on the epithelioid histology and tuberous sclerosis association. Am J Surg Pathol. 2009;33:289–97.

Blanco LZ, Schein CO, Patel T, et al. Fine-needle aspiration of metanephric adenoma of the kidney with clinical, radiographic and histopathologic correlation: a review. Diagn Cytopathol. 2013;41: 742–51.

Crapanzano JP. Fine-needle aspiration of renal angiomyolipoma: cytological findings and diagnostic pitfalls in a series of five cases. Diagn Cytopathol. 2005;32:53–7.

He W, Cheville JC, Sadow PM, et al. Epithelioid angiomyolipoma of the kidney: pathological features and clinical outcome in series of consecutively resected tumors. Mod Pathol. 2013;26:1355–64.

Horwitz CA, Manivel JC, Inampudi S, et al. Diagnostic difficulties in the interpretation of needle aspiration material from large renal cysts. Diagn Cytopathol. 1994;11:380–3.

Katz LB, Ehya H. Liesegang rings in renal cyst fluid. Diagn Cytopathol. 1990;6:197–200.

Kulkarni B, Desai SB, Dave B, et al. Renal angiomyolipomas: a study of 18 cases. Indian J Pathol Microbiol. 2005;48:459–63.

Kumar N, Jain S. Aspiration cytology of focal Xanthogranulomatous pyelonephritis: a diagnostic challenge. Diagn Cytopathol. 2004; 30:111–4.

Kuroda N, Toi M, Hiroi M, et al. Review of metanephric adenoma of the kidney with focus on clinical and pathobiological aspects. Histol Histopathol. 2003a;18:253–7.

Mai KT, Yazdi HM, Perkins DG, et al. Fine needle aspiration biopsy of epithelioid angiomyolipoma. A case report. Acta Cytol. 2001;45:233–6.

Raso DS, Greene WB, Finley JL, et al. Morphology and pathogenesis of Liesegang rings in cyst aspirates: report of two cases with ancillary studies. Diagn Cytopathol. 1998;19:116–9.

Shannon BA, Cohen RJ, de Bruto H, et al. The value of preoperative needle core biopsy for diagnosing benign lesions among small, incidentally detected renal masses. J Urol. 2008;180:1257–61.

Todd TS, Dhurandhar B, Mody D, et al. Fine needle aspirations of the cystic lesions of the kidney. Morphologic spectrum and diagnostic problems in 41 cases. Am J Clin Pathol. 1999;111:317–28.

Renal Cell Carcinomas

Abern MR, Tsivian M, Polascik TJ, et al. Characteristics and outcomes of tumors arising from the distal nephron. Urology. 2012;80:140–6.

Al Nazer M, Mourad WA. Successful grading of renal-cell carcinoma in fine-needle aspirates. Diagn Cytopathol. 2000;222:223–6.

Assad L, Resetkova E, Oliveira VL, et al. Cytologic features of renal medullary carcinoma. Cancer. 2005;105:28–34.

Auger M, Katz RL, Sella A, et al. Fine needle aspiration cytology of sarcomatoid renal cell carcinoma: a morphologic and immunocytochemical study of 15 cases. Diagn Cytopathol. 1993;9:46–51.

Caraway NP, Wojcik EM, Katz RL, et al. Cytologic findings of collecting duct carcinoma of kidney. Diagn Cytopathol. 1995;13:304–9.

Cheville JC, Lohse CM, Zincke H, et al. Sarcomatoid renal cell carcinoma: an examination of underlying histologic subtype and an analysis of associations with patient outcome. Am J Surg Pathol. 2004;28:435–41.

Delahunt B, Eble JN. Papillary renal cell carcinoma: a clinicopathologic and immunohistochemical study of 105 tumors. Mod Pathol. 1997;10:537–44.

Delahunt B, Sika-Paotonu D, Bethwaite PB, et al. Grading of clear cell renal cell carcinoma should be based on nucleolar prominence. Am J Surg Pathol. 2011;35:1134–9.

Ficarra V, Martignoni G, Maffei N, et al. Original and revised nuclear grading according to the Fuhrman system: a multivariate analysis of 388 patients with conventional renal cell carcinoma. Cancer. 2005;103:68–75.

Gilani SM, Tashjian R, Qu H. Clear cell papillary renal cell carcinoma with characteristic morphology and immunohistochemical staining pattern. Pathologica. 2012;104:101–4.

Huo L, Sugimura J, Tretiakova MS, et al. C-kit expression in renal oncocytoma and chromophobe renal cell carcinomas. Hum Pathol. 2005;36:262–8.

Klatte T, Streubel B, Wrba F, et al. Renal cell carcinoma associated with transcription factor E3 expression and Xp11.2 translocation. Incidence, characteristics, and prognosis. Am J Clin Pathol. 2012; 137:761–8.

Kuroda N, Toi M, Hiroi M, et al. Review of sarcomatoid renal cell carcinoma with focus on clinical and pathobiological aspects. Histol Histopathol. 2003b;18:551–5.

Layfield LJ. Fine-needle aspiration biopsy of renal collecting duct carcinoma. Diagn Cytopathol. 1994;11:74–8.

Liu J, Fanning CV. Can renal cell oncocytoma be distinguished from renal cell carcinoma on fine-needle aspiration specimens? A study of conventional smears in conjunction with ancillary studies. Cancer. 2001;93:390–7.

Liu Q, Galli S, Srinivasan R, et al. Renal medullary carcinoma: molecular, immunohistochemistry, and morphologic correlation. Am J Surg Pathol. 2013;37:368–74.

Masoom S, Venkataraman G, Jensen J, et al. Renal FNA-based typing of renal masses remains a useful adjunctive modality: evaluation of 31 renal masses with correlative histology. Cytopathology. 2009;20:50–5.

Nayar R, Bourtsos E, DeFrias EV. Hyaline globules in renal cell carcinoma and hepatocellular carcinoma. A clue or a diagnostic pitfall on fine-needle aspiration? Am J Clin Pathol. 2000;114: 576–82.

Ono K, Nishino E, Nakamine H. Renal collecting duct carcinoma. Report of a case with cytologic findings on fine needle aspiration. Acta Cytol. 2000;44:380–4.

Owens CL, Argani P, Ali SZ. Mucinous tubular and spindle cell carcinoma of the kidney: cytopathologic findings. Diagn Cytopathol. 2007;35:593–6.

Peyromaure M, Misrai V, Thiounn N, et al. Chromophobe renal cell carcinoma: analysis of 61 cases. Cancer. 2004;100:1406–10.

Qi J, Shen PU, Rezuki WN, et al. Fine needle aspiration cytology diagnosis of renal medullary carcinoma: a case report. Acta Cytol. 2001;35:735–9.

Radhika S, Bakshi A, Rajwanshi A, et al. Cytopathology of uncommon malignant renal neoplasms in the pediatric age group. Diagn Cytopathol. 2005;32:281–6.

Renshaw AA, Granter SR. Fine needle aspiration of chromophobe renal cell carcinoma. Acta Cytol. 1996;40:867–72.

Sarode VR, Islam S, Wooten D, et al. Fine needle aspiration of collecting duct carcinoma of kidney: report of a case with distinctive features and differential diagnosis. Acta Cytol. 2004;48:843–8.

Schinstine M, Filie AC, Torres-Cabala C, et al. Fine-needle aspiration of an Xp11.2 translocation/TFE3 fusion renal cell carcinoma metastatic to the lung: report of a case and review of the literature. Diagn Cytopathol. 2006;34:751–6.

Shen SS, Truong LD, Ayala AG, et al. Recently described and emphasized entities of renal neoplasms. Arch Pathol Lab Med. 2007;131:1234–43.

Simsir A, Chhieng D, Wei XJ, et al. Utility of CD10 and RCCma in the diagnosis of metastatic conventional renal-cell adenocarcinoma by fine needle aspiration biopsy. Diagn Cytopathol. 2005;33:3–7.

Srigley JR, Delahunt B. Uncommon and recently described renal carcinomas. Mod Pathol. 2009;22:S2–23.

Wang HY, Mills SE. KIT and RCC are useful in distinguishing chromophobe renal cell carcinoma from the granular variant of clear renal cell carcinoma. Am J Surg Pathol. 2005;29:540–6.

Wang S, Filipowicz EA, Schnadig VJ. Abundant intracytoplasmic hemosiderin in both histiocytes and neoplastic cells: a diagnostic pitfall in fine-needle aspiration of cystic papillary renal cell carcinoma. Diagn Cytopathol. 2001;24:82–5.

Wiatrowska BA, Zakowski MF. Fine-needle aspiration biopsy of chromophobe renal cell carcinoma and oncocytoma: comparison of cytomorphologic features. Cancer. 1999;87:161–7.

Small Round Cell Tumors

Das DK. Fine-needle aspiration (FNA) cytology diagnosis of small round cell tumors: value and limitations. Indian J Pathol Microbiol. 2004;47:309–16.

Iyer VK, Kapila K, Agarwala S, et al. Wilms' tumor. Role of fine needle aspiration and DNA ploidy by image analysis in prognostication. Anal Quant Cytol Histol. 1999;21:505–11.

Kumar R, Gautam U, Srinivasan R, et al. Primary Ewing's sarcoma/primitive neuroectodermal tumor of the kidney: report of a case diagnosed by fine needle aspiration cytology and confirmed by immunocytochemistry and RT-PCR along with review of the literature. Diagn Cytopathol. 2012;40:156–61.

Portugal R, Barroca H. Clear cell sarcoma, cellular mesoblastic nephroma and metanephric adenoma: cytological features and differential diagnosis with Wilms tumour. Cytopathology. 2008; 19:80–5.

Ravindra S, Kini U. Cytomorphology and morphometry of small round-cell tumors in the region of the kidney. Diagn Cytopathol. 2005;32:211–6.

Serrano R, Rodrigues-Peralto JL, DeOrbe GG, et al. Intrarenal neuroblastoma diagnosis by fine-needle aspirations: a report of two cases. Diagn Cytopathol. 2002;27:294–7.

Shet T, Viswanathan S. The cytological diagnosis of paediatric renal tumours. J Clin Pathol. 2009;62:961–9.

Thomson TA, Klijanienko J, Couturier J, et al. Fine-needle aspiration of renal and extrarenal rhabdoid tumors. Cancer. 2011;119:49–57.

Weeks DA, Beckwith JB, Mierau GW, et al. Renal neoplasms mimicking rhabdoid tumor of kidney. A report from the National Wilms' Tumor Study Pathology Center. Am J Surg Pathol. 1991; 13:1042–54.

Hematopoietic Lesions

Ahuja S, Grover G, Jha AK, et al. Extramedullary hematopoiesis presented as solitary renal mass: a case report with review of the literature. Diagn Cytopathol. 2010;39:435–7.

Hunter S, Samir A, Eisner B, et al. Diagnosis of renal lymphoma by percutaneous image guided biopsy: experience with 11 cases. J Urol. 2006;176:1952–6.

Orucevic A, Reddy VB, Selvaggi SM, et al. Fine-needle aspiration of extranodal and extramedullary hematopoietic malignancies. Diagn Cytopathol. 2000;23:318–21.

Subhawong AP, Subhawong TK, Vandenbussche CJ, et al. Lymphoproliferative disorders of the kidney on fine-needle aspiration: cytomorphology and radiographic correlates in 33 cases. Acta Cytol. 2013;57:19–25.

Truong LD, Caraway N, Ngo T, et al. Renal lymphoma. The diagnostic and therapeutic roles of fine-needle aspiration. Am J Clin Pathol. 2001;115:18–31.

Immunohistochemistry

Carvalho JC, Thomas DG, McHugh JB, et al. p63, CK7, PAX8 and INI-1: an optimal immunohistochemical panel to distinguish poorly differentiated urothelial cell carcinoma from high-grade tumours of the renal collecting system. Histopathology. 2012;60:597–608.

Gokden N, Mukunyadzi P, James JD, et al. Diagnostic utility of renal cell carcinoma marker in cytopathology. Appl Immunohistochem Mol Morphol. 2003;11:116–9.

Gupta R, Balzer B, Picken M, et al. Diagnostic implications of transcription factor Pax 2 protein and transmembrane enzyme complex carbonic anhydrase IX immunoreactivity in adult renal epithelial neoplasms. Am J Surg Pathol. 2009;33:241–7.

Hes O, Michal M, Kuroda N, et al. Vimentin reactivity in renal oncocytoma. Arch Pathol Lab Med. 2007;131:1782–8.

Kobayashi N, Matsuzaki O, Shirai S, et al. Collecting duct carcinoma of the kidney: an immunohistochemical evaluation of the use of antibodies for differential diagnosis. Hum Pathol. 2008;39:1350–9.

Mai KT, Teo I, Robertson SJ, et al. Immunostaining as a diagnostic aid in cytopathologic study of upper urinary tract urothelial carcinoma. Acta Cytol. 2009;53:611–8.

Nakazawa K, Murata S, Yuminamochi T, et al. p16(INK4a) expression analysis as an ancillary tool for cytologic diagnosis of urothelial carcinoma. Am J Clin Pathol. 2009;132:776–84.

Skinnider BF, Amin MB. An immunohistochemical approach to the differential diagnosis of renal tumors. Semin Diagn Pathol. 2005; 22:51–68.

Truong LD, Shen SS. Immunohistochemical diagnosis of renal neoplasms. Arch Pathol Lab Med. 2011;135:92–109.

Zhai QJ, Ozcan A, Hamilton C, et al. PAX-2 expression in nonneoplastic, primary neoplastic, and metastatic neoplastic tissue. A comprehensive immunohistochemical study. Appl Immunohistochem Mol Morphol. 2010;18:323–32.

Zhou M, Roma A, Magi-Galluzzi C. The usefulness of immunohistochemical markers in the differential diagnosis of renal neoplasms. Clin Lab Med. 2005;25:247–57.

Molecular/Genetic Studies

Koul H, Huh J-S, Rove KO, et al. Molecular aspects of renal cell carcinoma: a review. Am J Cancer Res. 2011;1:240–54.

Roh MH, Dal Cin P, Silverman SG, et al. The application of cytogenetics and fluorescence in situ hybridization to fine-needle aspiration in the diagnosis and subclassification of renal neoplasms. Cancer Cytopathol. 2010;118:137–45.
Vieira J, Henrique R, Ribeiro FR, et al. Feasibility of differential diagnosis of kidney tumors by comparative genomic hybridization of fine needle aspiration biopsies. Genes Chromosomes Cancer. 2010;49:935–47.

Rhabdoid Tumor

Barroca HM, Costa MJ, Carvalho JL. Cytologic profile of rhabdoid tumor of kidney. A report of 3 cases. Acta Cytol. 2003;47:1055–8.
Wakely Jr PE, Giacomantonio M. Fine needle aspiration cytology of metastatic rhabdoid tumor. Acta Cytol. 1986;30:533–7.

Urothelial Carcinoma of Kidney Pelvis

Olgac S, Mazumdar M, Dalbagni G, et al. Urothelial carcinoma of the renal pelvis: a clinico-cytopathologic study of 130 cases. Am J Surg Pathol. 2004;28:1545–52.

Metastatic Neoplasms

Gattuso P, Ramzy I, Truong LD, et al. Utilization of fine-needle aspiration in the diagnosis of metastatic tumors to kidney. Diagn Cytopathol. 1999;21:35–8.

Chapter 6
Adrenal Glands

Introduction

The majority of adrenal lesions, masses, or cysts are incidentally detected during imaging studies performed for investigation of extra-adrenal diseases. Most of these "incidentilomas" are benign, nodular hyperplasias, or adenomas, but other nonfunctional cortical or medullary neoplasms, even rarely, metastatic neoplasms without known primary malignancies, can be detected. In most cases, the decision for the management of these patients (type of treatment or follow-up without treatment) can be made based on the size and other imaging characteristics. Small masses (<3 cm) are usually benign, and larger ones (>4 cm) are malignant, but small malignant and large benign neoplasms have been reported.

Fine Needle Aspiration (FNA)

The use of FNA in the diagnosis of adrenal lesions is usually limited to single adrenal masses in patients with extra-adrenal malignancy to determine the nature of the mass. Most FNAs are performed by ultrasound (US) or computed tomography (CT) guidance. Endoscopic ultrasound (EUS) guided FNAs, almost all done on the left adrenal gland, have also been used in recent years. On-site evaluation (OSE) of the specimen helps to obtain adequate samples and direct the

Y.S. Erozan and A. Tatsas, *Cytopathology of Liver, Biliary Tract, Kidney and Adrenal Gland*, Essentials in Cytopathology 18, DOI 10.1007/978-1-4899-7513-3_6, © Springer Science+Business Media New York 2015

material for ancillary studies as needed (see Chap. 2). Complications of FNA include hematoma in the adrenal gland and pneumothorax. A few cases of tumor seeding in the needle tract have been reported.

Cysts

Benign cysts of adrenal gland are rare. They can be pseudo-cysts, vascular or epithelial. Aspiration material contains macrophages, leukocytes, and benign epithelial cells as well as erythrocytes and hemosiderin-laden macrophages in hemor-rhagic cysts.

Nodular Cortical Hyperplasia and Cortical Adenoma

Most of the incidentally detected adrenal masses represent hyperplastic nodules or cortical adenomas. They can be func-tional or nonfunctional. Cytomorphology of hyperplastic nodules and adenomas, functional or nonfunctional, is similar and is presented together.

Cytomorphology:
Specimens are usually cellular and composed of uniform single cells, aggregates, and tissue fragments in varying pro-portions. Individual cells have round nuclei with smooth borders and finely vacuolated cytoplasm (Fig. 6.1). Scattered large cells with larger nuclei may be present (Fig. 6.2). Because of the fragile cytoplasm, bare nuclei in a "bubbly" background are commonly seen. In cellular specimens, aggregates of bare nuclei could be mistaken as small cell carcinoma (Fig. 6.3).

Key features:

- Cells with round uniform nuclei and finely vacuolated cytoplasm
- Bare nuclei in a background of lipid droplets

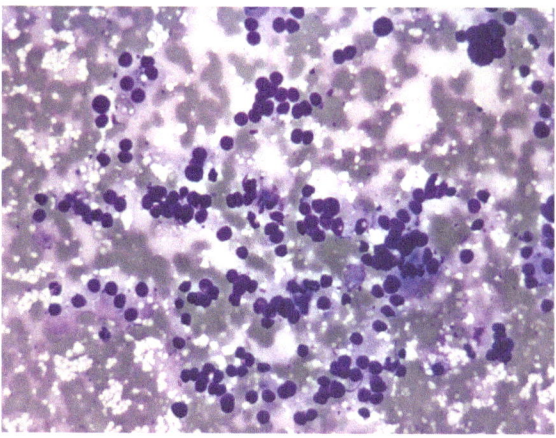

Fɪɢ. 6.1.   Adrenal cortical adenoma: Groups and single cells with round nuclei in a background of lipid vacuoles. Most cells have lost their cytoplasm or have ill-defined cytoplasmic borders. (Diff-Quik stain, medium power)

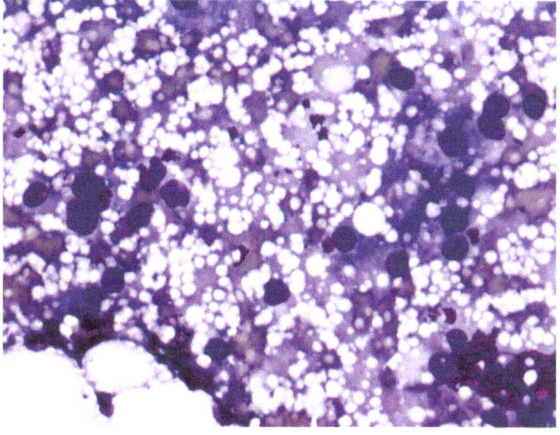

Fɪɢ. 6.2.   Adrenal cortical adenoma: Several cells with large nuclei. (Diff-Quik stain, high power)

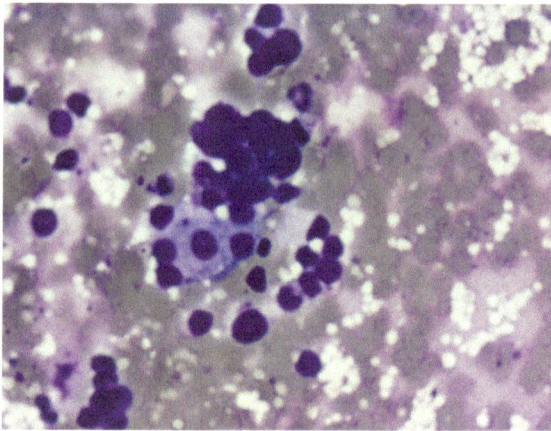

Fig. 6.3.   Adrenal cortical adenoma: Several tight groups of bare nuclei mimicking small cell carcinoma. (Diff-Quik stain, high power)

Differential diagnosis:
Benign proliferations of cortical cells, including adenomas, cannot be differentiated from adrenocortical carcinoma in FNA or core biopsy specimens. Metastatic tumors with clear cell features, specifically renal cell carcinomas and some hepatocellular carcinomas, may have similar morphologic features to those of adrenocortical neoplasms. Immuno-histochemical profile of these tumors helps to differentiate them from adrenal cortical neoplasms, which will be discussed under adrenal cortical carcinoma.

Myelolipoma

Myelolipoma is a rare benign tumor of adrenal gland usually found incidentally during abdominal imaging studies. They can reach large sizes. FNA provides a definitive diagnosis.

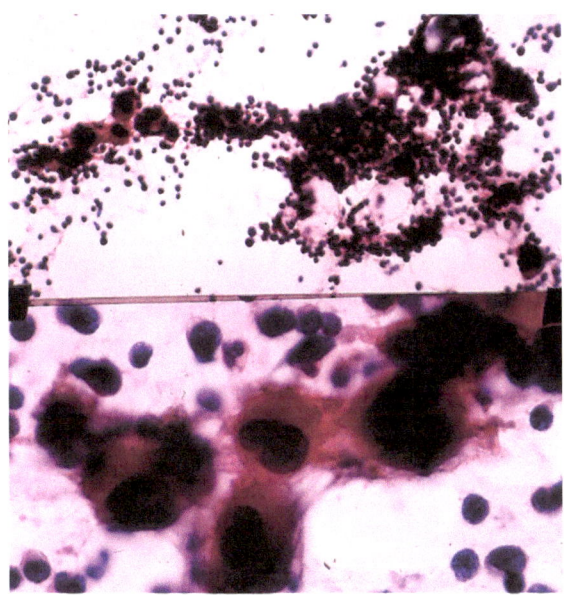

Fig. 6.4.   Myelolipoma: *Top*, mixture of adipose tissue and myeloid and lymphoid elements. (Papanicolaou stain, low power) *Bottom*, megakaryocytes. (Papanicolaou stain, high power). (*Top*) Published with permission from: Fine Needle Aspiration Cytology, eds. MK Sidawy, SZ Ali, Churchill Livingston/Elsevier, 2007, Chapter 10, Kidney and Adrenal Glands, YS Erozan, pages 299–346

Cytomorphology:
Characteristic findings are a mixture of fat tissue and hematopoietic cells. Erythroid, myeloid precursors, and megakaryocytes mixed with fat tissue or fat droplets are typically found (Fig. 6.4).

Key feature:

• Hematopoietic cells admixed with fat

Differential diagnosis:
In adequate samples, the cytopathological findings are quite specific. Extramedullary hematopoiesis may be considered in

the absence of fat tissue. The latter usually occurs at multiple sites and is associated with other conditions causing failure of hematopoiesis in bone marrow.

Pheochromocytoma

Pheochromocytoma is a rare neoplasm of adrenal gland arising from the chromaffin cells of the medulla. Over 90 % of the cases are sporadic. Familial cases belong to one of the multiple endocrine neoplasia (MEN) syndromes. Sporadic cases in adults are usually solitary masses.

The majority of pheochromocytomas are functional. Increased levels of vanillylmandelic acid (VMA) and catecholamines are found in the urine of about 90 % of patients with these tumors and are used in the diagnosis along with imaging studies. About 10 % of these tumors are malignant. In most publications, suspicion of pheochromocytoma is considered a contraindication for FNA because of the potential risk for hypertensive crisis and unstoppable bleeding. These complications, however, are rare; and FNA is performed in some cases, even if the possibility of pheochromocytoma exists. In these cases, it is recommended that the radiologist be prepared to deal with those complications.

Cytomorphology:
FNA general provides hypercellular specimens composed of single cells and loose cell groups. The tumor cells have varying morphology. Large pleomorphic cells, smaller neuroendocrine type cells, and spindle cells have been described. Binucleated and multinucleated cells and occasional intranuclear pseudoinclusions are present (Fig. 6.5a, b).

Immunohistochemistry:
Stains for NSE, synaptophysin, and chromogranin are positive (Fig. 6.6). S-100 stains sustantecular cells.

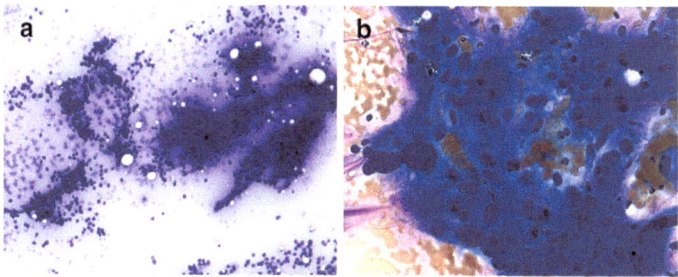

Fig. 6.5.   Pheochromocytoma: (**a**) Single cells and tissue fragments with uniform round or ovoid nuclei with ill-defined cytoplasm. Several rosette formations are present. (Diff-Quik stain, low power) (**b**) Syncytial appearing tissue fragment and single cells. Markedly pleomorphic nuclei. (Diff-Quik stain, high power)

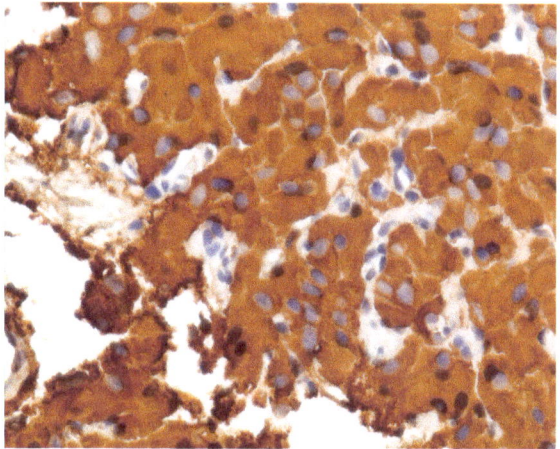

Fig. 6.6.   Pheochromocytoma: Strong positivity with Chromogranin stain. (Cell block, medium power)

Key features:

- Cellular specimens with single cells and loose groups of cells
- Large pleomorphic cells and smaller neuroendocrine-type cells
- Binucleated and multinucleated cells

TABLE 6.I.   Immunohistochemistry of neoplasms metastatic to adrenal glands.

Neoplasms	Positive immunostains
Lung	
Adenocarcinoma	TTF1, Napsin A
Small cell carcinoma	TTF1
Breast	ER, Mammoglobin, GCDFP, GATA3
Colon	CK20, CDX2
Stomach	CK20, CK7
Pancreas	CK 19-9
Endometrium	ER, PR
Ovary, serous	WT1, ER, PAX-8
Ovary, mucinous	CA 125, PAX-8
Renal cell carcinoma	RCC, Vimentin, CD10, PAX-8, PAX-2
Melanoma	S-100, Melan A, HMB45, SOX-10, MITF

Differential diagnosis:
The main differential diagnoses include adrenocortical carcinoma, sarcomatoid renal cell carcinoma and, rarely, retroperitoneal sarcoma. Immunohistochemical stains are usually needed for differentiating pheochromocytoma from the others (Table 6.1).

Adrenocortical Carcinoma

Adrenocortical carcinoma is an extremely rare tumor, mostly found in persons between 40 and 50 years of age. The tumor is usually very large (average 16 cm), however, tumors measuring less than 6 cm have been reported. Adrenocortical carcinoma is a very aggressive tumor with a poor prognosis. Small size is considered the most reliable feature for a better outcome. The majority of the tumors (85–90 %) are functional. Histologically, the tumor has varying patterns and cellular features, most of which can be seen in some benign cortical neoplasms. Local invasion or distant metastasis is criteria for the definitive diagnosis of malignancy in these tumors. Several systems (e.g., Weiss System) based on multiple histopathological parameters have been used for evaluating

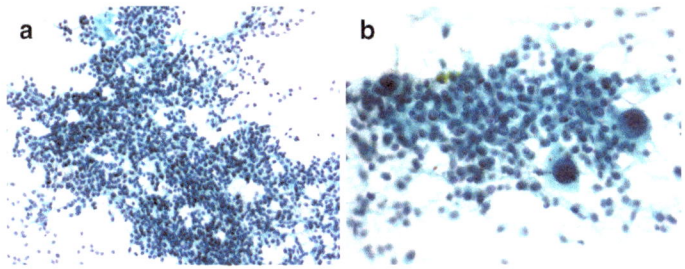

FIG. 6.7.   Adrenal cortical carcinoma: (**a**) Large cellular tissue fragment composed of predominantly uniform small cells with rosette formations. (Papanicolaou stain, low power) (**b**) The tissue fragment from the same tumor also has rosette formations, but larger nuclei with coarser chromatin and multiple nucleoli. Two cells next to the fragment have extremely large, hyperchromatic nuclei. (Papanicolaou stain, medium power)

adrenocortical malignancy with reliable results in resected tumors. In small tissue or FNA specimens, this evaluation cannot be made accurately because of the small sampling.

Cytomorphology:
FNA specimens are usually very cellular. Morphology ranges from well-differentiated to poorly differentiated forms. Tumor cells appear singly, in loose groups, or tissue fragments. They have hyperchromatic nuclei and dense cytoplasm (Fig. 6.7a). Very large single cells with gigantic nuclei among the smaller cells can be seen (Fig. 6.7b).

Poorly differentiated tumors exhibit marked pleomorphism with bizarre nuclei (Fig. 6.8) and tissue fragments of pleomorphic cells with sarcomatous features (Fig. 6.9). The oncocytic variant of adrenocortical carcinoma has granular eosinophilic cytoplasm similar to oncocytoma.

Immunohistochemistry:
Immunohistochemical stains are positive for inhibin-alpha, calretinin, synaptophysin, melan A, and CAM 5.2. Chromogranin A and PAX-8 are usually negative. HMWCK is negative.

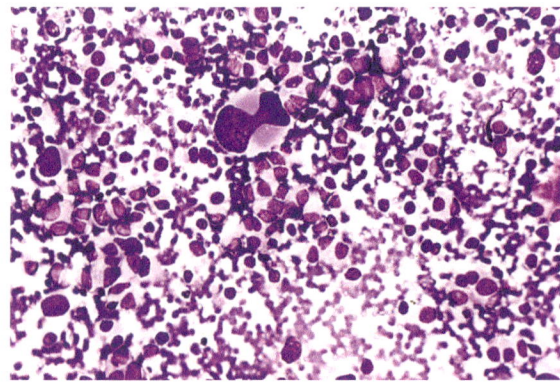

FIG. 6.8. Poorly differentiated adrenal cortical carcinoma: Predominantly single cells with pleomorphic nuclei. Note the gigantic atypical nucleus. (Diff-Quik, medium power)

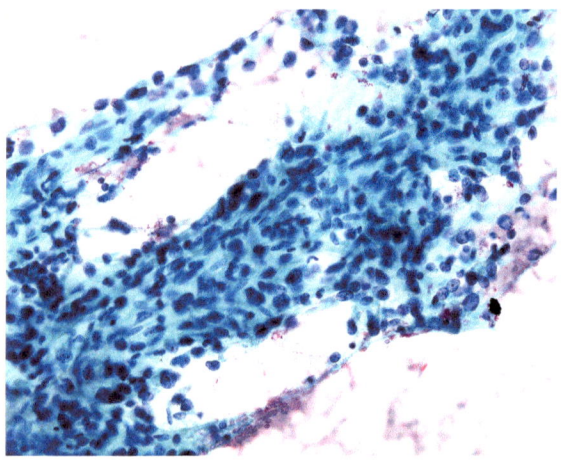

FIG. 6.9. Poorly differentiated adrenal cortical carcinoma: A tissue fragment of tumor. Note the oval, round, and spindle shaped pleomorphic nuclei. (Papanicolaou stain, medium power)

Key features:

- A rare malignant neoplasm
- Usually large tumor (more than 6 cm)
- Majority are functional
- Tumor cells have varying degree of differentiation
- Marked nuclear pleomorphism with giant nuclei can be seen
- Mitoses, including atypical ones, and necrosis can be seen
- Immunostain for inhibin alpha, calretinin, melan A, CAM 5.2, and synaptophysin is positive. Chromogranin and HMWCK are negative

Differential diagnosis:

Because of the wide range of cytomorphology of adrenocortical carcinomas, both some primary and metastatic tumors are included in the differential diagnosis. ACC cannot be differentiated from cortical adenoma in FNA specimens. Other neoplasms included in the differential diagnosis are pheochromocytoma, renal cell carcinoma, hepatocellular carcinoma, clear cell carcinoma of the ovary and uterus, malignant melanoma, and large cell carcinoma of the lung. Immunohistochemical stains are usually needed for the differential diagnosis. There are a series of immunostains which help to differentiate these neoplasms. Adrenal 4 binding protein (Ad4BP) or SF-1 is reported to be very effective in differentiating ACC. Ad4PB/SF1 reactivity was shown in almost all tumor cells in ACC, but in none of the other neoplasms listed above.

Neuroblastoma

Neuroblastoma is one of the most common tumors of childhood following leukemias, lymphomas, and brain tumors. Most occur in children under the age of 5 years. Adrenal is the most common site. Age and stage are the most significant prognostic factors. About one-third of the tumors are in an advanced stage with metastases to lymph nodes, bone, liver,

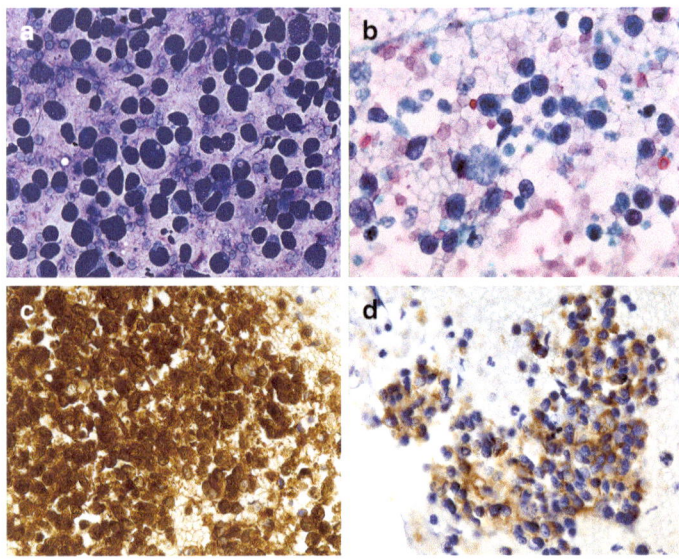

FIG. 6.10.   Neuroblastoma: (**a**) Single cells slightly varying in size with large nuclei and generally very scant cytoplasm. (Diff-Quik stain, high power) (**b**) Tumor cells. Scant to moderate amount of cytoplasm and single or multiple small nucleoli. (Papanicolaou stain, high power) Immunostains: (**c**) Neuron-specific enolase (NSE), (**d**) Chromogranin, all positive. (**c** and **d**, medium power)

and lung. Neuroblastomas, especially in children under 1 year of age, may mature and transform into ganglioneuroma.

Cytomorphology:
FNA specimens are hypercellular, composed of small cells appearing singly or in groups with occasional rosette formations (Homer-Wright rosettes). Tumor cells have round to ovoid nuclei and a thin rim of cytoplasm. Occasional cells with more cytoplasm and eccentric nuclei and cells with elongated nuclei and unipolar cytoplasmic extension may be present (Fig. 6.10a). Nuclei can be hyperchromatic or show an evenly distributed granular chromatin pattern. Foci of nuclear molding can be seen. Fine granular and fibrillary material (called neuropil) is present in the background (Fig. 6.10b).

Tumors differentiating to ganglioneuroma have increasing numbers of ganglion cells having large nuclei with reticular chromatin and prominent nuclei.

Immunohistochemistry:
Tumor cells react to neuroendocrine markers including NSE (Fig. 6.10c), chromogranin (Fig. 6.10d), and synaptophysin and microtubule-associated proteins (MAP1 and MAP2).

Key features:

- Common tumor in children occurring generally under the age of 5 years
- Cellular specimen with single cells and groups
- Tumor cells with round to oval nuclei and scant cytoplasm
- Rosette formations, some with fibrillary centers (Homer-Wright rosettes)
- Fine granular and fibrillary material (neuropils) in the background
- Varying number of ganglion cells in different stages of differentiation to ganglioneuroma

Differential diagnosis:
Other small round cell neoplasms, mainly nephroblastoma, large-cell and Burkett lymphomas, Ewing sarcoma, primitive neuroectodermal (ES-PNET) and small cell desmoplastic tumors should be included in the differential diagnosis. Immunohistochemical stains are needed in most cases to establish the specific diagnosis.

Metastatic Neoplasms

Adrenal glands are a frequent site of metastatic carcinomas. Metastasis is usually unilateral, but bilateral involvement has been reported in up to 49 % of cases. Adenocarcinomas are the most common type of cancers to metastasize to adrenal. Lung and breast make up the majority of metastatic cancers in most published series, followed by gastrointestinal tract, pancreas, and kidney. Hepatocellular and bile duct

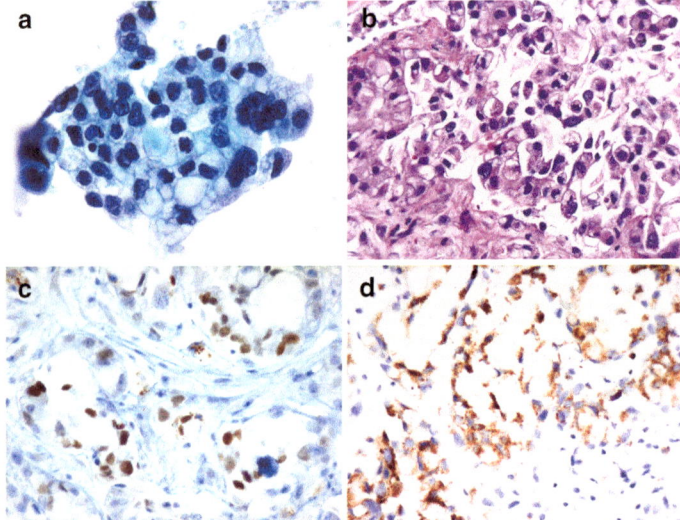

FIG. 6.11.   Metastatic adenocarcinoma, primary lung: (**a**) A large tissue fragment composed of disorganized tumor cells with pleomorphic nuclei. Intracytoplasmic vacuoles, several acinar formations, and luminal borders (*upper edge of the fragment*) indicate glandular differentiation. (Papanicolaou stain, medium power) (**b**) Same tumor. (Cell block, H&E stain, medium power) (**c**) Positive nuclear staining with TTF-1, medium power (**d**) Positive cytoplasmic staining with Napsin A, medium power.

carcinomas have been found in higher numbers of cases in East Asian countries. Examples of several metastatic cancers are shown in Figs. 6.11a–d, 6.12, 6.13, and 6.14.

Lymphoma can be primary or secondary to systemic lymphoma (Fig. 6.15).

Immunohistochemical stains are needed for the differential diagnosis and/or confirmation of the primary site (Table 6.1).

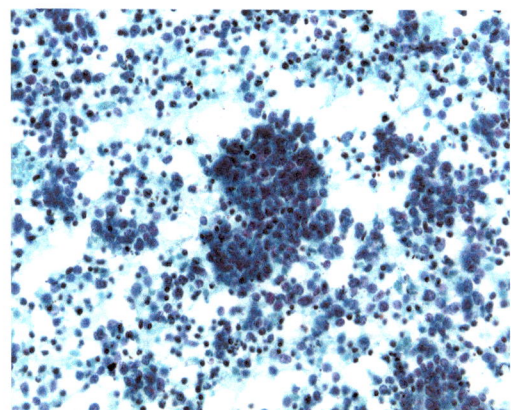

FIG. 6.12.   Metastatic small cell carcinoma: Tissue fragments and single cells. Small cells with scant cytoplasm and nuclear molding. (Papanicolaou stain, medium power)

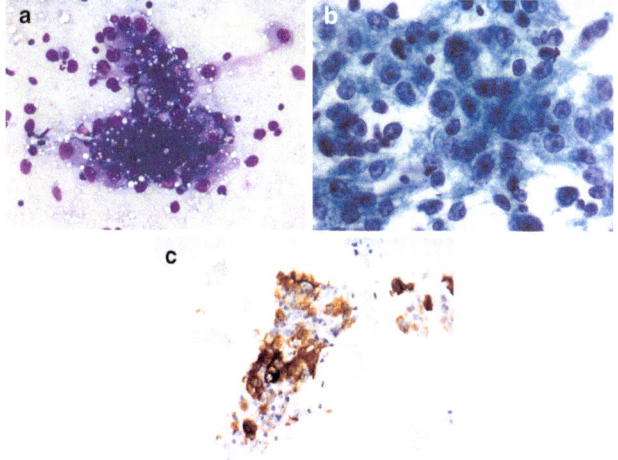

FIG. 6.13.   Metastatic hepatocellular carcinoma: (**a**) Large cells with round nuclei and vacuolated cytoplasm. This morphology is similar to that of adrenal cortical carcinoma. (Diff-Quik stain, medium power) (**b**) Note large nuclei with macronucleoli which are typical of hepatocellular carcinoma. (Papanicolaou stain, high power) (**c**) Immunostain HepPar is positive confirming hepatic origin. (Medium power)

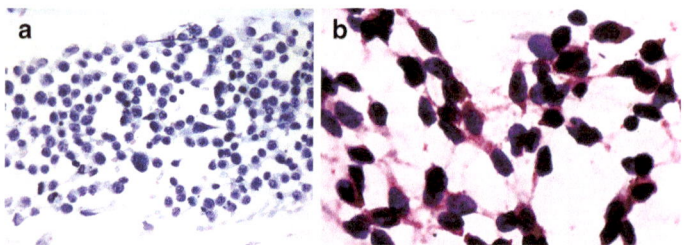

FIG. 6.14.   Metastatic melanoma: Single cells having large nuclei with prominent nucleoli. The cells are rounded or have unipolar cytoplasmic extensions. (**a**) (Papanicolaou stain, medium power) (**b**) (HMB45 immunostain, high power). (**a**) Published with permission from: Fine Needle Aspiration Cytology, eds. MK Sidawy, SZ Ali, Churchill Livingston/Elsevier, 2007, Chapter 10, Kidney and Adrenal Glands, YS Erozan, pages 299–346.

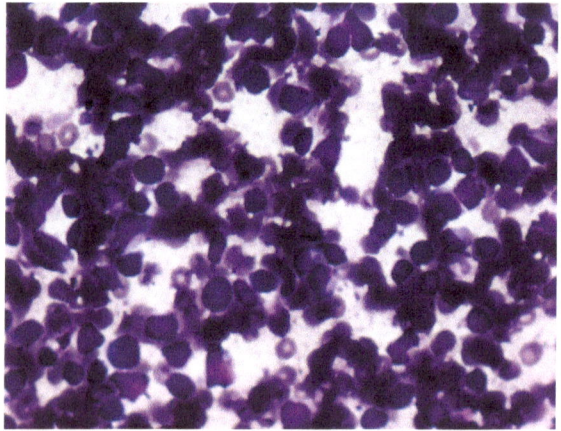

FIG. 6.15.   Large B-cell lymphoma: Single cells with large round nuclei and scant cytoplasm in a background of erythrocytes. Flow cytometry in this case confirmed the diagnosis. (Diff-Quik, high power)

Suggested Reading

General: FNA

de Agustin P, Lopez-Rios F, Alberti N, et al. Fine-needle aspiration biopsy of the adrenal glands: a ten-year experience. Diagn Cytopathol. 1999;21:92–7.

Erozan YS. Kidney and adrenal glands, Chapter 10. In: Sidawy MK, Ali SZ, editors. Fine needle aspiration cytology. Philadelphia: Churchill Livingston/Elsevier; 2007. p. 299–346.

Geisinger KR, Stanley MW, Raab SS, et al. Adrenal. In: Modern cytopathology. New York: Churchill Livingstone Elsevier; 2004. p. 619–42.

Lumachi F, Borsato S, Brandes AA, et al. Fine-needle aspiration cytology of adrenal masses in noncancer patients: clinicoradiologic and histologic correlations in functioning and nonfunctioning tumors. Cancer. 2001;93:323–9.

EUS-Guided FNA

DeWitt J, Alsatie M, LeBlanc J, et al. Endoscopic ultrasound-guided fine-needle aspiration of left adrenal gland masses. Endoscopy. 2007;39:65–71.

Eloubeidi MA, Black KR, Tamhane A, et al. A large single-center experience of EUS-guided FNA of the left and right adrenal glands: diagnostic utility and impact on patient management. Gastrointest Endosc. 2010;71:745–53.

Jhala NC, Jhala D, Eloubeidi MA, et al. Endoscopic ultrasound-guided fine-needle aspiration biopsy of the adrenal glands: analysis of 24 patients. Cancer. 2004;25:308–14.

Stelow EB, Debol SM, Stanley MW, et al. Sampling of the adrenal glands by endoscopic ultrasound-guided fine-needle aspiration. Diagn Cytopathol. 2005;33:26–30.

Uemura S, Yasuda I, Kato T, et al. Preoperative routine evaluation of bilateral adrenal glands by endoscopic ultrasound and fine-needle aspiration in patients with potentially resectable lung cancer. Endoscopy. 2013;45:195–201.

Adrenal Cysts

Sebastiano C, Zhao X, Deng F-M, et al. Cystic lesions of the adrenal gland: our experience over the past 20 years. Hum Pathol. 2013; 44:1797–803.

Myelolipoma

Porcaro AB, Novella G, Ficarra V, et al. Incidentally discovered adrenal myelolipoma. Report on 3 operated patients and update of the literature. Arch Ital Urol Androl. 2002;74:146–51.
Settakorn J, Sirivanichai C, Rangdaeng S, et al. Fine-needle aspiration cytology of adrenal myelolipoma: case report and review of the literature. Diagn Cytopathol. 1999;21:409–12.

Pheochromocytoma

Jimenez-Hefferman JA, Vicandi B, Lopes-Ferrer P, et al. Cytologic features of pheochromocytoma and retroperitoneal paraganglioma: a morphologic and immunohistochemical study of 13 cases. Acta Cytol. 2006;50:372–8.
Niveditha SR, Suguna BV, Krishnamurthy, et al. Cytologic features of malignant cystic pheochromocytoma: a case report. Acta Cytol. 2007;51:200–2.
Shidham VB, Galindo LM. Pheochromocytoma. Cytologic findings on intraoperative scrape smears in five cases. Acta Cytol. 1999; 43:207–13.

Adrenocortical Carcinoma

Aubert S, Vacrenier A, Leroy X, et al. Weiss system revisited. A clinicopathologic and immunohistochemical study of 49 adrenocortical tumors. Am J Surg Pathol. 2002;26:1612–9.
Ren R, Guo M, Sneige N, et al. Fine-needle aspiration of adrenal cortical carcinoma: cytologic spectrum and diagnostic challenges. Am J Clin Pathol. 2006;126:389–98.
Sangoi AK, Fujiwara M, West RB, et al. Immunohistochemical distinction of primary adrenal cortical lesions from metastatic

clear cell renal cell carcinoma: a study of 248 cases. Am J Surg Pathol. 2011;35:678–86.

Sasano H, Suzuki T, Moriya T. Recent advances in histopathology and immunohistochemistry of adrenocortical carcinoma. Endocr Pathol. 2006;17:345–54.

Weissferdt A, Phan A, Suster S, et al. Adrenocortical carcinoma: a comprehensive immunohistochemical study of 40 cases. Appl Immunohistochem Mol Morphol. 2014;22:24–30.

Index

Y.S. Erozan and A. Tatsas, *Cytopathology of Liver, Biliary Tract, Kidney and Adrenal Gland*, Essentials in Cytopathology 18, DOI 10.1007/978-1-4899-7513-3, © Springer Science+Business Media New York 2015